Genocide by Denial

How Profiteering from HIV/AIDS Killed Millions

T0269621

Peter Mugyenyi

FOUNTAIN PUBLISHERS
Kampala

Fountain Publishers
P. O. Box 488
Kampala - Uganda
E-mail: sales@fountainpublishers.co.ug
           publishing@ fountainpublishers.co.ug
Website: www.fountainpublishers.co.ug

Distributed in Europe and Commonwealth countries
outside Africa by:
African Books Collective Ltd,
P. O. Box 721,
Oxford OX1 9EN, UK.
Tel/Fax: +44(0) 1869 349110
E-mail: orders@africanbookscollective.com
Website: www.africanbookscollective.com

Distributed in North America by:
Michigan State University Press
1405 South Harrison Road
25 Manly Miles Building
East Lansing, MI 48823-5245
E-mail: msupress@msu.edu
Website: www.msupress.msu.edu

ISBN 978-9970-02-753-8

Privacy Policy

Careful consideration has been given to safeguard individual privacy.
Accordingly, unless the information was already in public domain or
voluntary consent was first obtained, no real names or specific identities of
patients alive or dead have been used. Also, some details of events that may
apparently lead to public exposure of individuals have been changed without
altering the essential facts of the story.

Dedication

*This book is dedicated
to the memory of all people who died of AIDS.
Singled out for special remembrance are millions of
men, women and children who would have lived, but died
simply because they were too poor to pay the
price of the life-saving drugs.*

Over 40 million infected with HIV virus;
The vast majority are African in their prime,
Of which 25 million are dead and still counting…..
8000 deaths per day.
Yet these deaths are not inevitable!

ℤℤ ℤℤ ℤℤ

"Obu niburwaireki oburikwita omushaija,
bukataho omukazi n'abaana enju bakagisiba? Pe!

Translation: "What kind of a monster disease is this that kills a man,
his wife and all their children, thus closing the entire homestead?"

Yudesi Ndimbirwe,
Author's mother, 1989

Contents

Acknowledgements

I can't possibly thank all the people who helped me in my work in the area of AIDS, which is the basis of this book. However, I would like to first of all thank my family, especially my children: Jimmy, Fred, Michelle, Denise, and Martin. I sincerely thank Ernest Rusita, for his mentorship and good advice. I am indebted to Liz Paren, for taking time to review the first draft and making useful suggestions. I thank Mark Harrington for his encouragement, and David Blumenkrantz, for his advice. I am also grateful to Lera Munati for urging me to pick up the pen, and Anthony Canavan for his help in shaping the book.

For a variety of reasons I acknowledge with thanks and gratitude the following people: Ben Mbonye, Jesse Kagimba, Gregg Gonsalves, Amy Cunningham, Rob Cunane, Sam Rwakojo, Fred Makoha, Mohamed Kibirige, and Ceppie Merry. I am also greatly appreciative of Tony Fauci, and Mark Dybul for their role in changing the AIDS situation in Africa from one of gloominess and desperation to one of hope and optimism.

I am greatly indebted to all my colleagues at the Joint Clinical Research Centre, Kampala, especially Samson Kibende, Cissy Kityo, Francis Ssali, Stefano Tugume, John Oloror, Rose Byaruhanga, Mary Mulindwa, Santrina Batto, to mention but a few for standing shoulder to shoulder with me during the most difficult times, when we jointly tried to find ways and means of finding a solution to the AIDS scourge in Uganda. Whatever I may have achieved would never have been possible without their help and participation

I reserve my very special thanks to all my patients, first and foremost, because they are the reason that I am a doctor. I thank especially all those that were affected or infected by HIV/AIDS for their patience and resilience despite the pain of it all, while faced with this century's most vicious plague and denial of help. It is my sincere hope that this record will contribute to the deliverance of future patients faced with similar diseases of mass devastation.

Lastly I recognize with due respect the vital role that President Yoweri Museveni played in the control and treatment of AIDS in Uganda. Most importantly I thank him for his timely intervention and leadership which helped to save numerous lives. His foresight and strategic vision in starting the JCRC created the opportunity for me to add my humble contribution.

Peter Mugyenyi
Kampala
2008

Introduction

It was just unthinkable!

Even in their wildest dreams, no resident of the sleepy rural south western Ugandan district of Rakai could have possibly imagined that this mystifying new affliction, which cropped up insidiously in their midst way back in 1980, would metamorphose into arguably the most catastrophic tragedy in the entire human history.

"Was it a curse, witchcraft, or a disease?" the bamboozled villagers wondered.

Nobody could figure out exactly where it came from and why it crept in to spoil the usually quiet village life of Kasensero, and neighbouring areas. The usual daily highlights were the early morning wake-up cockerel call, and the ravving engine noises of heavily-loaded long distance trucks that frequently made overnight stops in the area's small trading centres on their way from the coastal ports to the neighbouring countries. However, in time, putting one and one together, the mystified inhabitants increasingly discerned an emerging pattern among the victims. They first noticed that the mysterious affliction seemed to be confined to only a few scattered locations in the district. Then they increasingly noticed that it appeared to choose some particular persons, who adopted certain peculiar lifestyles. The early sufferers were by and large relatively well-off by the village standards. The poor, who were the vast majority, initially escaped almost unscathed. These observations were quite reassuring for everyone else outside the perceived vulnerable group, who for a little while thought they were out of harm's way. But alas, this ray of hope was soon dimmed, as the rude intruder turned on its head.

With increasing alarm, the villagers discovered that in reality, contrary to earlier observations, the queer disease affected persons of different walks of life. But the worse was still to come. For when the initially nameless disease exploded onto the general public, leaving a trail of blood the entire community froze in terror. No one felt safe any more. Then whispers started about a curse and bad omen hovering over the area. Terror stirred up the community, and inevitably there was a frantic counter-reaction that brought out the community health watchdogs in full strength. They included witchdoctors, herbalists, various religious leaders, spiritual healers and Western doctors, all fretfully trying to find a remedy. New and descriptive names for the lethal plague were coined based on the observed signs and symptoms the tortured victims suffered before they invariably succumbed. Inexorably, the death toll rose from a mere trickle to hundreds, then on to thousands, to hundreds of thousands - and still counting, as the scourge spread ruthlessly, eventually reaching all parts of the country.

When the connection was confirmed between penetrative sex and the new disease, and that all victims inevitably died, then a new form of torment was added to the awful physical pain in the form of stigma fuelled by sheer terror. Stigma made the already dreadful situation of the victims worse - much worse. Sufferers hid from the prying eyes of the public but not always successfully. In some cases they could not even share their predicament with friends and family, mainly because they feared rejection. Many affected families wrapped their hands around their faces in "shame". Holier-than-thou religious leaders preached about unrepentant sinners being responsible for the scourge. Victims sought solace and salvation of a different kind from the many new religious sects that sprang up specifically to assuage or just exploit the desperation.

When the disease that started among the relatively well-to-do entered the peasant and poverty-stricken populations it found a fertile breeding-ground which, right from the beginning, guaranteed mayhem. It defied even the most ingenious scientific interventions, and relentlessly unfolded into mankind's most catastrophic pandemic in living memory. By late 1980's, the situation in Uganda had seriously deteriorated bearing the hallmark of a gruesome genocide in the making. As the modern day Grim Reaper that Ugandans dubbed *slim*, but which the rest of the world came to know as Acquired Immune

Deficiency Syndrome (AIDS), tortured and killed children, and adults alike - more especially the poor - I was right there, not only as a witness but also as one who tried to do something about it. It presented me with enormous challenges, yet like everyone else I had no inkling of how to go about it. But I still took it on regardless.

As I started on the task, I soon discovered that AIDS was not just a disease or simply one of the most sophisticated medical and scientific challenges. Among other things, it was a hot, contentious international problem, which stretched beyond a mere disease process, or its prevention and treatment. I was to learn that AIDS was a complex humanitarian, moral, ethical, social, economic, psychological, cultural, legal, and political crisis of immense magnitude with diverse implications. In fact, AIDS directly or indirectly touched on virtually all aspects of life of almost everyone in Sub-Saharan Africa. With regard to treatment, access which should have been a top priority, I was appalled to find that it was being denied to millions of people who needed it for their very survival on account of their poverty. The sheer carnage presented a clear moral imperative for all urgent humanitarian response and the immediate mobilisation of resources to address the emergency. To my suprise however, the rich countries turned a blind eye to the disaster. The increasingly devastated poor countries were abandoned to their fate. Yet if the rich countries had reacted immediately, this monster disease could have been nipped in the bud especially in areas where it had not taken a firm hold. Quite the reverse, the rich world just stood by as millions perished excruciatingly - until it was far too late. The most shocking lesson that I learned was that most of the dreadful suffering and deaths were not necessarily inevitable. In fact, millions of lives could have been saved, thus averting the very worst of the catastrophe. But this required the rich and mighty countries to act resolutely in unison. Yet no rich country's finger was lifted. The hard-heartedness of the world's rich towards the plight of the resource-constrained countries at the time of their greatest need dumbfounded me. It emerged that so many lives did not really mean much as long as they were poor.

I was to learn that the awesome pharmaceutical multinational industry or *The Big Pharma,* as it is widely known, is one of the most powerful forces in the world, over and above being one of the most lucrative businesses on earth. The proprietors are fully determined to cling to their huge profits and monopoly at almost any cost. In their business, human suffering and disasters are not their priority concern. From personal experience, I was to learn that merely trying to obtain life-saving drugs for dying patients could have gotten me a long jail sentence. Indeed, more often than not, victims of diseases are viewed like any other lucrative business opportunity. The Big Pharma's enormous authority and formidable lobby extends to the corridors of the world powers. They influence countries and world trade policies that impact directly on virtually each and every person on earth on an almost daily basis. To challenge their vast power is just like a bird kicking the ocean.

Working with my colleagues at the Joint Clinical Research Centre (JCRC) and with other partners of many nationalities, I tried all that I could, under very difficult circumstances, to help alleviate mankind's most heartrending catastrophe. However, all the efforts seemed to be in vain. Then my campaign had a rather unexpected boost when out of the blue I was invited to the US Congress, to make a presentation about the catastrophe of AIDS in Africa. Then in totally unforeseen circumstances I was summoned back to Washington, and ended up being grilled by the US government special committee as I tried to convince them to come to the assistance of the AIDS-devastated African continent. In January 2003 I was fighting eviction by the powerful landlord of my humble AIDS treatment clinic and research laboratory, housed in an old royal prime minister's residence on the outskirts of Kampala, when suddenly I was invited as a special guest of the wife of the most powerful man on earth, the President of the United States.

Although I can now see a glimmer of hope in the current initiatives, I have no doubt that genocide most foul, mainly by denial, was committed and continues to date at a lower but still devastating level. The carnage was allowed to go overboard, under the cover of the current TRIPS

(Trade Related Aspects of Intellectual Property Rights), patents laws and World Trade Organisation (WTO) regulations, that authorised the Big Pharma to maintain monopoly rights on the life-saving drugs that made them too costly - out of reach of the poor.. Meanwhile, the United Nations, especially the rich countries, failed to act with the urgency and generosity that the terrible situation cried out for, until the stink of it all reached them in the bastions of their privileged circumstances far away from the wretched of the earth. The facts of the disaster are self-evident. According to UNAIDS, an estimated 25 million people had by 2006 been killed by AIDS, including 2.8 million who died in 2005 alone. The AIDS catastrophe has demonstrated so much that is tragically wrong with the current world order, which allowed genocide of this magnitude to happen – legally! In the meantime, the nightmare lives on as AIDS continues on its devastating march torturing and killing far too many people, especially the very poor

Meanwhile the rich world has not committed enough funds, and has not made right policies and laws to save humanity from this century's most devastating catastrophe. Instead the current half-hearted measures merely afford the disease a chance to further metamorphose into a new form of reinvigorated disaster. I fear the worst because I still do not see any serious international measures or new laws in the pipeline. Clearly, the AIDS catastrophe demonstrated the danger inherent in the current TRIPS agreement in which protection of profits far outbalances the imperative to protect human lives. This sad situation calls for an urgent review of TRIPS, patents and WTO laws, aimed at the removal of all ambiguities and gimmicks so as to resolutely establish an ethical platform for vigorously addressing humanitarian emergencies, including diseases of mass destruction. Sadly, instead of overhauling the fraudulent laws, some powers and special interest groups have instead recommended only some minor amendments. The proposed changes are not even robust enough to solve the current AIDS crisis and therefore have no chance of protecting humanity, especially the poor in future disasters.

The remaining hope for the world, especially the poor people, is the inherent goodness within humanity that must recapture the higher moral ground in critical issues that affect the health and well-being of all. Humanity, if we are to understand it in its true meaning, cannot have it any other way.

1
Ingredients of a disaster

The Gathering Storm

The very first seeds of a new and mysterious disease must have been sown by the mid-1970s, or more likely earlier, in Uganda's south-western district of Rakai, which borders Tanzania. It could have started on either side of the border or even in neighbouring Congo, but no one is really sure. Perhaps it is not so important now, despite so much "udo" about the issue. Rakai is situated about 190 km from Uganda's capital, Kampala. Although Rakai is a multi-tribal district, the dominant tribes are the *Baganda* and the *Banyankole,* but it also include tribes of Rwandan origin, and various other ethnic groups from both Uganda and Tanzania. In 1982, it was in this same district in a place called Kasensero that the first diagnosed Ugandan cases of AIDS originated. Since then Rakai District has been devastated by AIDS to such an extent that some households were completely erased by the epidemic.

However, in retrospect, it was not until early 1980 that the residents clearly discerned a weird and horrifying new illness in their midst. It looked like some curse had descended on the sleepy rural district, leaving every inhabitant bewildered and terrified. Mathias Mugisha, a Ugandan investigative and feature journalist, reported that when a parish chief of Bugera village, Luanda Sub-county in Rakai, came down with a strange illness in 1980, the villagers whispered that he was bewitched. By the time of his death, the chief had lost his hair and nails, a phenomenon that the villagers had never witnessed before. Since the village extends to the Tanzanian Bukoba district boundary, the villagers thought the witchcraft had been unleashed from across the border. However, a scattering of similar cases had also occurred on the other side of the border, and the Tanzanians in turn blamed the Ugandans for the curse. The weird disease almost started a small war.

Daggers drawn, the Ugandans and Tanzanians accused each other of witchcraft.

The witchcraft curse was initially dubbed *Juliana* after the brand name of popular low cost but trendy clothes, which Ugandan businessmen used to sell in the border markets. The relatively prosperous *Juliana* traders and a number of youths wearing T-shirts with Juliana labels were among the first to succumb to the new plague. The matter became so serious that it brought the cross-border trade to a virtual standstill. Some superstitious villagers burned items from this trade, including cash and household goods. A few prosperous ones even set their own cars on fire. To their dismay, however, the spell was not appeased and the dreadful deaths just continued. Exorcism and counter witchcraft rituals were tried out but when even these failed, the terrified villagers fled from the markets where they suspected the witchcraft originated. The then booming Rukuyu market on the Ugandan side of the border with Tanzania was abandoned and has never recovered.

Rakai district was named after the main town in the area of the same name, which together with another town, Lyantonde, were popular overnight stops for long-distance drivers from the coastal towns of Mombasa in Kenya and Dar es Salaam in Tanzania, on their long journey across Uganda to Congo, Rwanda and Burundi. Commercial sex workers facing tough economic conditions under Idi Amin's regime, and some other women finding it hard to put food on the table, found a ready and lucrative business with the high-spending truck drivers. The nearby relatively prosperous fishing communities, especially Kasensero and some parts of Kakuuto on the shores of Lake Victoria, were not very easily accessible, because of the swamps and poor access roads. The roads were hardly passable during rainy seasons, yet these areas were among the first to be afflicted by the new disease. Poor accessibility served the people of the area well by concealing one of the area's main occupations. It was a bustling smuggling hub for goods from Kenya and Tanzania across Lake Victoria in canoes to the lucrative Ugandan market, which was facing severe shortages as a result of Amin's mismanagement of the economy. The relatively well-off smugglers and fishmongers would move with their booty from the shores to the nearby towns of Rakai and Lyantonde to join in the bonanza.

There is a common belief that truck drivers might have introduced AIDS into inland Rakai from the coast, and this may be true though there is no definite evidence. However, their major contribution, as far as could be reasonably determined, was to transport HIV in their trucks along the trade route. Later, after 1982, when HIV surveys were carried out, it was found that the rates were highest in Rakai and declined with increasing distance in both directions. This does not imply that Rakai was the origin, any more than that the homosexual communes in California were the origin of AIDS. More likely, it was merely the conducive conditions in the area that favoured and then nurtured the initial localised outbreaks.

With regard to the long-distance drivers, a small study done in 1999 in Rakai found a staggering 33 % of truck drivers and 67 % of barmaids were infected with HIV. M. Gysels, R. Pool and K. Bwanika studied the sexual characteristics of truck drivers in an effort to elucidate their role in the AIDS saga. Their findings are revealing as to why this group was particularly prone to HIV. The popularity of roadside stops depended on easy access to sex, among other considerations like accommodation and food. Many of the truck drivers, especially during the scarcity of virtually all goods during the Amin era, were also smugglers who brought various, high-demand goods into the area to sell. Some local petty traders depended on this trade for survival, and formed alliances with truck drivers. Smuggling was a serious crime in Uganda under laws introduced by Amin. The penalty for smuggling could be as severe as facing a firing squad. In fact, some people suffered exactly that. Therefore, it was imperative to associate with trusted middlemen to provide extra security to truckers. In addition, the alliance between truckers and middlemen provided an important service in connecting truck drivers to commercial sex workers. The sex workers were not always so obvious as there was no "Red light district". In fact, the barmaids were the ones that doubled up as prostitutes. The sex middlemen knew the local women well and were sometimes given a stipend by the women to find them business. Some of the middlemen would become agents of some of the very women they already had sex with themselves. The money the truck drivers got from selling smuggled goods paid for the prostitutes and accommodation, and the balance went into booze in the plentiful bars in the town. Buying alcohol for the prostitutes was a well-recognised pick-up strategy. Other cash-laden people were the middlemen who made profits from the goods bought from truckers, the smugglers from Kasensero fish landing villages, the traders and fishermen. These were the ones that frequented the bars, and could afford both the high cost of beers and payment for the services of prostitutes. In the late 1970's and early 1980's condom use was virtually unknown in Rakai. The prostitutes and the well-to-do that were in the centre of it all were among the first victims.

Whenever people fell sick they returned to their home villages to die, and the villagers noticed that sufferers almost always wasted away, failed to respond to any medical treatment and inevitably died. On account of the pattern of emaciation of the victims, *Slim* was the name coined by the rural people of Rakai displacing *Juliana* as the name of the new plague. Being slim or suffering sudden weight loss from whatever cause came to be equated with a bad omen, - a sign of imminent death.

When AIDS was later defined, Slim and AIDS became synonymous. Other names in local languages including "ukimwi" in Swahili and "mukenenya" in one of Uganda's languages - Luganda - were coined much later.

By the end of 1981, the situation had deteriorated, bearing all the hallmarks of a catastrophe in the making, though very few recognised it as such. As the disease affected more people, even the elders could not recall a similar malady either in living memory or from their ancestor's ancient tales, apart from one dubious ailment in the past. Some old people in the villages could vaguely recall an outbreak of a wasting disease perhaps in the early 1920s, which seemed to have somehow fizzled out as mysteriously as it appeared. Some few old surviving traditional healers talked of the tubers of some wild plants, which had been used successfully to treat this disease. Some elderly women led teams of youths to the few remaining forests in the hunt for the mysterious plants. Some were found, but no one could guarantee that they were the exact ones used in the earlier outbreak or that it actually had worked. However, when the tubers were tried on the victims of the new disease there was no discernible effect.

Meanwhile, several hundred kilometres from Rakai in another small town of Naluwerere, in eastern Uganda about fourty kilometres from the Uganda–Kenya border crossings of Malaba and Busia, people were also struck by a puzzling disease that had also mysteriously cropped up. It bore a striking resemblance to the Rakai outbreak but nobody immediately made the connection. Besides the strange disease there was little else in common between the two areas. The two communities belonged to different tribes, spoke different languages, and were culturally and otherwise different in many ways. Understandably, any linkage would not immediately become clear. However, like Rakai, this particular town was also a popular overnight stop for long-distance truck drivers on their journey from Mombasa. The trucks that cleared the border customs late found the small town, close to the slightly larger one of Bugiri, very convenient for an overnight stay. From the mid-1970's, Idi Amin had issued a decree banning all heavy vehicles from travelling at night in Uganda. It was said that Idi feared a military coup, and could not risk heavy trucks carrying military personnel and arms in surprise night movements to depose him. Amin's decree remained in force until 1979 when he was overthrown; this helped the spread of HIV as truck drivers were by decree forced to make overnight stops. No truck driver could risk breaking this strict order. It would mean losing all the merchandise and, worse still, their lives at the hands of Amin's undisciplined army and rampaging thugs. The town offered some sort of security to the drivers despite the fact that some of Amin's soldiers used to extort money from the truckers ostensibly to provide security, and this was very preferable to outright robbery, which was the only alternative. Secondly, the drivers and turn boys on the trucks would take turns to consort with the many sex workers, in their trucks or in the town lodges.

Early the next morning the trucks would set off, travelling very slowly on the badly potholed roads on the long journey to Congo, Rwanda and Burundi. The evening curfew would find them in Rakai. There they would resume the practice of the previous night. On the return leg after delivering the payload, the same routine would resume.

At about the same time, thousands of kilometres away in Los Angeles, the mainly white gay community were also startled by the outbreak of a rare form of fatal pneumonia that was on a steep rise among the sexually active. In addition, a very rare cancer called Kaposi's sarcoma, not previously endemic in United States, had started cropping up in the same group, mainly of gay young men, at the ages when these conditions would be extremely rare. No one at the time could have imagined any linkage between these two events in two totally diverse communities and environments. Besides, the affected Rakai populations were, as far as could be ascertained, exclusively heterosexual. Yet across the oceans in the USA, the heterosexuals seemed to be spared. The Americans, like the Ugandans, were puzzled about the possible causes and origin of the mysterious disease. Some saw it as divine retribution. The gay community, finding themselves in a corner, mobilised and pulled together and up to now remain some of the most vocal AIDS activists in the world.

It was not until June 5, 1981, that the United States' Centres for Disease Control and Prevention (CDC) made some headway. This was followed by the issuing of its first warning about the outbreak of a rare pneumonia. However, it was not until the following year that the mystery was better explained by linking the pneumonia to the newly-defined Acquired Immune Deficiency Syndrome, or AIDS, as it is known today.

The Rude Welcome Home

What was to turn out to be my long involvement in the struggle against AIDS, started as soon as I disembarked from an old Uganda Airline Boeing 707 one October afternoon in 1989. I felt a strange uneasiness. Something was not quite right. To begin with, I was supposed to be feeling great, because I was finally returning home, sweet home, from a long exile. Instead I found the humour and tempo of the good old vibrant and cheerful people that I once knew rather cowed. The welcome hugs were not quite as intimate as they used to be and the smiles no longer spontaneously warm. If it were not for the familiar Ugandan multi-tribal faces and varied accents, the same old Entebbe airport terminal building - still unmistakable despite the grime, cobwebs all over the soot covered ceiling, dry cracked paint on the walls and non-functioning luggage conveyors - I would have been forgiven for thinking that I had landed at a foreign airport. Clearly a bad omen hovered in the air, but I could not immediately discern the cause.

As I travelled along the forty kilometre obstacle course that passed for a road, from the airport to Kampala, I was taken aback by the devastation my country had suffered during my long absence. What should have been an exultant ride home instead turned out to be a scary, uncomfortable experience. I was to learn later that some potholes were real bomb craters courtesy of the Tanzanian artillery, which inflicted the damage during the 1979 war as they repulsed and retaliated against Amin's invading forces. Amin met his Waterloo in a misadventure that could be likened to a modern version of fighting windmills, when he marched into Tanzanian Kagera district seeking to annex it.

As we drove towards Kampala, I sat holding on tightly to the broken door handle of the old Toyota taxi that should have long been condemned to scrap. Oncoming taxis in a race to pick up passengers along the way sped towards us making a head on crash seem unavoidable, only to veer off at the moment. Surprisingly, our driver, did not seem unduly perturbed and never reached for the car horn to warn of danger. As a fresh returnee from Jeddah, Saudi Arabia, where almost everyone is a car horn user, this incongruous calm in the face of apparent danger was amazing.

As we entered the outskirts of the once beautiful legendary seven hills city of Kampala, I could see desolation and ruin almost everywhere. The most booming business was the gruesome trade in death. There prominently displayed by the roadside was an abundant and varied assortment of coffins. I could see that business was brisk, as several pickup trucks were busy loading the merchandise. I could also see carpenters busy in the workshops assembling more coffins.

As I settled in, it soon became clear that this was just a brief glimpse of the daily horror and agony suffered by my fellow countrymen, as a result of AIDS. I was soon to find out that the AIDS scourge had propelled Uganda to the unenviable rank of the most AIDS affected country in the world. Yet my medical training in Uganda, and the considerable experience I had acquired in several countries abroad, had not prepared me for the most complex infectious disease in history, that leaped far beyond medicine, into international geopolitics, religion, commerce, racism, human rights and beyond.

The Baptism of Fire

It was almost thirteen years that had elapsed since I fled Mulago Hospital, Kampala's National Referral and Teaching Hospital, at the height of Idi Amin's tyranny. On my return to Uganda, and Mulago Hospital, I found enormous changes - almost all of them for the worse.

Way back on 2 February 1977, after my escape, I had arrived in Lesotho fleeing from Mulago Hospital because of insecurity and unbearable conditions, to start what turned out to be twelve years of exile. In Lesotho, my first home away from home, I worked as a medical officer at the Queen Elizabeth II Hospital in the capital, Maseru, where I stayed for two years, and then moved on to Britain in 1979. I finally ended up in Saudi Arabia where, ironically, I was to come face to face with Idi Amin in person, the very one I had run away from. Fleeing from Amin's Uganda was a very risky undertaking. I was smuggled out of the country by two old friends Ireneo Namboka, who later worked for the United Nations, and Jack Sabiti who became a politician. I was whisked away lying low in the back seat of Jack's Volkswagen. If we had been caught, we would have been extremely lucky to escape with our lives. To me, or indeed any other escapee, it was a journey of no return as long as Amin remained in power. I went into exile to face an uncertain future, armed only with my medical degree and a determination to work hard.

Lesotho was a wonderful place for a young medical graduate to practice. I loved the people, the work and the country, also known adoringly as the *Kingdom in the sky* because of its mountainous terrain. The hospital was very busy with endless queues of patients with all kinds of medical problems, but there was a severe shortage of doctors. However, I was very much thrilled by the resultant hard work, because it provided me with plenty of opportunities for hands-on practice in virtually all medical and surgical disciplines. Indeed, I accumulated considerable experience, which helped my career development.

From Lesotho I moved to Britain, which offered better postgraduate training and job prospects. I first undertook a clinical attachment that was essential for all foreign medical graduates, in the north-eastern town of Sunderland. My immediate boss was the elderly Dr Haycock, who always wore a three piece, striped, navy blue suit and, who to us was as close to a god as can be imagined. The purpose of the clinical attachment was, first of all, to assess whether the entrant was conversant with the English language, secondly to determine whether he had the necessary skills and was of acceptable medical standards. Successful candidates would then be recommended for employment within the National Health Service. Satisfying all requirements under the awesome Dr Haycock was not easy. The other doctors that I found there warned me right from the beginning that life would be really tough. Under no circumstances, I was warned, was I to talk out of turn in his presence or even address him unless he first talked to me. There was no need to know his first name because there were no circumstances under which anyone would dare address him by it or even say it out loud. I broke all the cardinal rules, but certainly not on purpose. I was just being myself. Surprisingly, old Haycock did not seem to mind at all and instead seemed to enjoy it. I rather liked the grandfatherly Haycock, because I appreciated and shared his concern for the welfare of the sick little children that were topmost priority in his work. Somehow there was a connection between us because he went out of his way to make sure that I was promptly paid my allowance of £40 a week, and he also arranged with the hospital administration to allow me use of the room after the official period of my attachment, while he helped me get a permanent job. I was told he had never done this for anyone else. He generously commended my work and was to write a very good recommendation for me, which gave me the best possible start and laid a good foundation which ensured that I was never out of a job all the time I was in the UK.

My first fully-paid job in the UK was at Newcastle Hospital paediatric heart section where for the first time I encountered new technologies for children's heart diagnosis and treatment. Pat, one of the senior nurses, went out of her way to make our difficult work and lives even harder. Our duties as junior doctors included taking blood samples for special tests from the babies and putting up intravenous drips. Finding blood vessels in the tiny limbs of the little ones, especially the pre-term babies, was a very delicate piece of work that Dr Paoulos, my colleague, and I were quite good at but unfortunately Pat, one of the senior nurses constantly disrupted our work. Whenever the babies whimpered in pain, as was inevitable, she would say we were hurting them. Yet, if there were any delay in taking the blood she would be the first to complain. Soon we noticed that these unreasonable complaints only happened when a particular senior doctor was around. We therefore devised a method of getting around her by skipping the coffee break, which she would never miss because the fancied doctor hardly ever missed his coffee too. At the best of times, the work of junior doctors in UK - was very busy and involved working very long hours. However, the practice was rewarding. Most senior doctors and nurses were highly professional, considerate and supportive. Challenged by the demanding work, we all pulled together, supported each other by sharing out the heavy workload even if it meant being on duty twenty-four hours. In hindsight, it all seems rosy, and certainly the gruelling work and close supervision made the UK hospitals among the very best training institutions for any young doctor. On top of the heavy schedule, I successfully combined it with rigorous postgraduate training in Paediatrics. I was rewarded with regular promotions that saw me rise through the ranks to the fairly senior position of Registrar in Swansea, South Wales. My superiors in Swansea were Doctors Agarwal, Forbes and Evans, who recommended me for further promotion. When the

Saudi Arabian Government advertised for experts from Britain to work in their country, they were reluctant to let me go because they had earmarked me for promotion. However, when I consulted Mr Ernest Rusita a former Uganda ambassador to Russia and the UK, then in exile in London, he advised me otherwise, urging that the Saudi Arabian offer was a more senior position which promised much better professional opportunities for advancement. It was an agonising decision for me to take, but in 1984 I accepted the post of a consultant Paediatrician, and set off with my wife, Christine, and four year old daughter, Michelle, for a new life in Saudi Arabia.

Our arrival in Saudi Arabia in March 1984 was rather unreceptive. We first landed in Jeddah but had to proceed to the capital Riyadh to first report to the Ministry of Health headquarters. I expected an interview or some sort of introduction to my new work in the kingdom. There was nothing of the sort. The Ministry of Health official did not even utter a word, but just wrote something in Arabic on a piece of paper which he handed to me, and then gestured that he had finished with me. I did not know what the note said and what to do with it. As I waited in the corridor puzzled, other recruits I had travelled with from London, an Irish man and an Indian doctor, joined me. We were all at sea, and asked anyone that passed by whether they spoke English, without success. Finally, a technical officer emerged from an office, collected all the documents and read to us what was written. The three of us had been posted to Jeddah. He handed me tickets for my family and we left for the airport. Back in Jeddah I found I had to pay for our own accommodation, although in London we were told by the Saudi embassy that the moneyed Saudi government would cover all expenses until we were well settled. In Jeddah we again had to report to the regional Ministry of Health headquarters for posting. There I met an amazing racist official, an Egyptian by the name of Hassan, whose job it was to welcome the expatriates and put them on the payroll. The salary rates in our case were fixed in London according to qualifications and level of expertise. Hassan promptly signed off the white doctor, but the Indian and I were set aside. Turning to the Indian doctor first he told him that there was a mistake in his salary scale.

"As an Indian your salary cannot be the same as a European," he said, "You either accept an Indian salary scale or go back where you came from. We shall of course pay for your ticket back. Do you accept or not?" Hassan demanded.

"Yes" replied the tired Indian doctor resignedly. He had a wife and two young tired and fretful children, and the long wait in Riyadh, the round trip, and the unexpected expenses, were just too much for him. He just wanted to get a respite from it all. Accordingly, Hassan proceeded to slash his salary on paper and inserted new terms, which the luckless doctor promptly signed, and left for his new work post. Then it was my turn. As he turned to me, I did not wait for him to ask the question. I told him right away that I did not accept any terms other than those I agreed to in London. "In that case you have to go." Hassan was livid with anger. "Who do you think you are anyway? You just saw the Indian accept his salary level and you have the impudence to say that you cannot accept yours? Look," he said as he pulled out a document in Arabic, which was presumably the official salary scales, "they mistakenly gave you the European scale in London. In this country, Africans are supposed to be on this scale" he said pointing to a line on a document that I could not read.

"Excuse me, sir, I have seen an English translation of the same official document in London. It talks only about qualifications not race," I explained.

"Do you think you know my work better than me?" he retorted. "Either you accept the new salary scale or you go back. I will give you the ticket back right away if you so decide. The choice is yours and you have to choose right now," he added without even looking up, assuming that I would go ahead and sign the documents. He filled in the new salary and presented the form to me for signature.

"No sir," I told him. "I am going back."

For the first time, I saw him hesitate. Hassan was in fact not the one who made the final decisions about salaries and tickets. His posturing perhaps made him feel more powerful than he really was because decisions to do with money were under the tight control of Saudi nationals only, whose big offices were upstairs on the top floor. To get my ticket approved Hassan needed to ascend to the big officers who wielded real authority. Something about this task seemed to bother him, and he just asked me to take a seat while he continued to go about his chores of processing documents of various junior officials. Hours later after an agonising wait, Hassan finished the queue, and I was relieved expecting that my ordeal would soon be over. However, he just ignored me and proceeded to his tea break and a hearty chat with the other workers. His occasional gesture towards my direction and the muted laughter, suggested that the group were being entertained by Hassan's quips at my expense. It was late in the afternoon and I was tired. I walked over to the group and told Hassan rather impatiently, that I wanted my ticket and passport back so that I could go.

"Everyone else has accepted the new terms. You have to accept that you are not a European." Hassan's cohort burst into giggling laughter as he went on to admonish me. "If you sign the papers you will be fine. You know you can't get the salary I am offering you in your poor Africa." Hassan insisted.

I was hungry and angry. I was therefore finding it extremely difficult to remain composed. "Don't waste any more of my time, sir, I need to move on," I said to him in a frustrated raised voice.

Luckily for me, the head of the Ministry, a kindly Saudi gentle giant of a man who was later introduced as Dr Jomjoom, happened to be on his way out, was attracted by the noise and came to enquire. Hassan tried in vain to stop me from talking to him but I quickly explained my ordeal. He beckoned Hassan and me, to follow him back to his office. On our way up I shared an elevator with Hassan as Dr Jomjoom ascended alone. I was amazed by Hassan's dramatic chameleon act! He suddenly became cheerful and considerate man, and referred to me as his very good friend. When we got to Dr Jomjoom's huge office, Hassan kept signalling that I should keep quiet and let him explain things. He had, however, pushed me a step too far, and despite my usual patience and resilience, it looked to me then that I would not make it in Saudi with the likes of Hassan, and I therefore just wanted out. However Dr Jomjoom, a German trained surgeon turned administrator, was of a different calibre. He apologised for the excesses of his official and confirmed that my London contract terms were correct and proceeded to approve the salary. He subjected the crestfallen Hassan to a harsh tongue lashing in Arabic. I learnt later that Hassan's contract was not renewed, thus ensuring future recruits a much softer landing.

As I did not go with enough money, I had to move my family out of the unaffordable hotel to an abandoned government flat without air conditioning. The heat was unbearable, and my daughter and wife were not holding out well. We fled from the premises, and took refuge in the house of Dr Frederick and Josephine Makoha who were kind enough to host us until I was paid my first salary after a long wait, and moved into a place of our own. Dr Makoha, a Ugandan, who had earlier been signed up from the UK, was already well established in his job of a consultant gynaecologist in the same hospital. A couple of months later, the unsettling situation improved, and Ernest's assessment seemed to come true. I was appointed the head of Paediatrics and quickly got engrossed in the rigours and routine of one of Jeddah's busiest government hospitals.

Saudi Arabia was a very curious place to live and work. One hears much about the harsh conditions, the restrictions and the highly bureaucratic system, yet as far as medical practice was concerned they had some good hospitals and funds to make the dreams of any clinician come true. As the kingdom was short of manpower, almost all nurses and the vast majority of doctors were foreigners. However, at work and outside, the red tape and restrictions tended to get on virtually every foreigner's nerves. One had to always be very careful that no laws, written or otherwise, were violated because minor infringements could lead to unpleasant consequences. However, on the positive side the salaries were reasonable and tax-free. The ordinary Saudi people and most Saudi colleagues were very pleasant, kind and hospitable. I was able to advance well professionally, and certainly appreciated the time I spent there despite the rude landing. It was also in Saudi Arabia that I saw my very first laboratory tested and confirmed AIDS case, which I would have missed if it were not for a circular from the Ministry of Health issued to all health facilities in the kingdom.

The different kind of harsh conditions that I encountered on my return to Uganda did not entirely take me unawares, because I was quite prepared. I had kept my ears to the ground keenly following developments at home and therefore had a fairly reasonable anticipation of what I could fnd on the ground. I managed to put aside some modest savings over time, to support my family on return. I was therefore fairly prepared to endure the hardships in order to serve my country. This strategy was later to pay dividends, as my initial government monthly salary was so small that I had to wait a whole year for it to accumulate so as to be worthwhile before I collected it. Even then, it was only enough to sustain my family of four for a couple of weeks. At the time my one-year's salary in Uganda was equivalent to a quarter of an equivalent expert's monthly salary in Saudi Arabia.

Reporting for work on my very first day, at good old Mulago Hospital, where I was posted as a Consultant Paediatrician, I ran into an old colleague who expressed great surprise to see me back.

"I am sorry that you were silly enough to return to this God-forsaken country," he said as he shook his head in disapproval, while we shook hands in greeting. "Welcome to the nightmare of AIDS," he said in a fake theatrical voice, as he curtsied. It was amazing that even in the midst of numerous deaths some people would still emerge with their sense of humour intact! "AIDS is exterminating our people. It is almost too unbearable to watch," he added sombrely. Winking mischievously, he warned, "As for the babes, just forget it. Don't even think about it." Shaking his head, again, he went on to say: "It's carnage everywhere. Terrible! Even our classmates have not been spared. Do you remember Steven? Barnard? …. All of them dead."

He went on to mention others in the pipeline of death, explaining that he could tell by the then well known signs of AIDS. Any lingering doubt I had was soon dispelled by the scenario that confronted me in the children's ward. Though I had geared myself psychologically for the worst, what I was to witness in the ward was shocking beyond my worst fears. It was a baptism of fire.

Until then, my experience with AIDS was very limited. In fact I failed miserably to diagnose the very first case of AIDS that I ever saw. In my defence, though, my peers at the time would not have fared any better, because this was back in 1981 when AIDS was still a mysterious illness. At that time a withered five year old Ugandan male was referred to me at Morriston Hospital in South Wales, UK, where I was working as a Paediatric Medical Officer. He was brought by a visibly ailing mother, having been directed to me by one of her relatives who lived in London. The mother told me of her child's long, painful and mysterious illness that had baffled all the numerous doctors in Uganda and Kenya whom she had run to in a desperate attempt to save her baby's life. The quest for a cure had finally led the resolute mother to the UK for more advanced medical tests and hopefully effective treatment as a last resort.

I was presented with a sad looking boy I call David, aged about six years but with the size of a two year old. He was scared of doctors, but with time seemed to be reassured because in our hospital children's doctors did not wear white coats, which to David were associated with painful injections. The mother reported that her child had just failed to thrive, and suffered from recurrent serious infections which either responded poorly to medical treatment or not at all. The child attracted much interest, among my colleagues as a diagnostic puzzle. Even the more senior colleague, a brilliant Irish clinician, the late William Forbes, was at sea like the rest of us. It would be many years later that I could put my finger on the correct diagnosis based on the information from the child's relatives, in a sort of historical oral post-mortem. I was told that the child's entire family consisting of two siblings and parents had all died! All had developed what is now easily recognisable as typical AIDS signs and symptoms. One by one the ailing parent, watched all the children, including David, die despite their frantic efforts to get them the best medical treatment. However, the parents died suddenly in a fluke car "accident", widely believed by many of their relatives to have been a double suicide.

I vividly remember my very first confirmed AIDS case. It is to me like one of those shocking "where were you events", such as the assassination of J. F. Kennedy, or 9/11, that seem to freeze in people's memory forever. However, I never thought that it would become my future occupation. In this situation, it was the case of a sickly, pathetic child by the name of Mustapha that I saw in Saudi Arabia in 1985. He was referred to me in Jeddah with signs and symptoms any medical professional in Uganda could have readily recognised as AIDS related, but then to my colleagues, and me, it was a brainteaser. Although we all knew about AIDS, the diagnosis did not immediately spring to mind, partly because AIDS was then said to be almost non-existent in the kingdom of Saudi Arabia. No doctor dared test anybody for HIV. It was taboo! Indeed Mustapha would have died undiagnosed if it had not been for a Saudi Ministry of Health circular referred to above that warned all doctors and especially the dentists, to be aware and protect against AIDS. The circular specifically warned that the most likely patients to have HIV were Africans. Therefore the warning in itself would not have resulted in Mustapha getting tested for HIV since he was Arab. Credit goes to the hospital director, Dr Ahmad Ashour, who took his cue and ordered the laboratory chief to spot check all the blood samples in the hospital laboratory for AIDS. He wanted this done in order to give him an idea of the scope of the problem in the hospital. Among the samples tested was Mustapha's.

The laboratory chief, a pleasant but rather nervous Pakistani technologist, came to my ward shivering despite the Saudi midday sauna temperatures, stammering that he wanted to see me "v-ve-very-very privately". Behind locked doors in my office, he told me the startling news that also solved a mystery for me.

"Your p-patient Mustapha has A-A-AIDS," he stammered almost in a whisper, glancing side to side as if to make sure that no one was listening. He handed me the laboratory report. "This is not the kind of news that you would like to take out of this room," he said nervously as he withdrew the laboratory report from my hands. "Now that you know, you have no need for this. It was for your eyes only." He said as he tore the report to pieces. As he headed for the door he suddenly seemed to remember something and paused. "A-And one more-more t- thing, d-do-doctor," the stammer was back, "we did not have this conversation," he concluded as he reached for the door key.

"No" I said just to reassure him, "We did not."
No mention, of course, was made of the results of the other samples that he had tested, but the petrified expression of the technologist did not encourage much optimism. He was obviously scared out of his wits by the AIDS stigma, and whatever else he had seen in his laboratory. To me that was a defining moment as far as AIDS was concerned. I had diagnosed my very first case! A week later Mustapha, the lovable child that had suffered a painful puzzling illness almost from birth, was dead.

That was the only experience I had had about AIDS as I started my new job in Mulago Hospital in 1990. However, the first battle I had to fight was not against AIDS; but it was serious enough to completely ruin my first day at my new workplace. When I reported to the new Mulago children's Ward 1C, where I had been posted by my new boss, Professor Charles Ndugwa, I was revolted to find the ward flooded with raw sewage. Incredibly I found a doctor in the midst of a ward round followed by five, medical students, himself seemingly oblivious to the stinking mess. I tiptoed to him, introduced myself, and asked why the ward was not either closed or cleaned up.

"You obviously do not live in this part of the world, do you?" he said. "Do you think we love this stuff? Anyway, don't mind; you will get used to it," he added dismissively, and not without a hint of irritation.

I went straight to the Nurse's office to check on the duty rota. As I found that I was off duty that day, I charged out of the ward and made a bee line for the estates department. There I found a wizened, bronzed, British expatriate, clad in khaki shorts, humming an old popular country song. I was informed that he was in charge of the hospital rehabilitation as part of British aid to Uganda. I briefly explained the terrible situation in Ward 1C, more specifically the nauseating stink, and then complained that I was finding it difficult to carry out my job because he had not done his part.

"I know conditions are hard for everyone but as an expert civil engineer, I am sure you can quickly fix it" Although I was boiling inside, I tried to be moderate, and humour him a little so that I could get his cooperation. As he just stared at me rather incredulously, without uttering a word, I laboured to elaborate, "Honestly it is not possible for me to work today but I will return early tomorrow morning expecting a clean ward" I added as I prepared to depart.

"You talk tough, man! Where the heck have you come from?" he finally opened his mouth. He turned out to be a very humorous man when I got to know him later.

"Let's leave the tough talk for tomorrow- that is if I find the ward still in a mess," I replied, as I stormed out of his office, leaving him behind making funny faces.

Early the next day, I found the ward clean, with a fresh smell of *jik*. However, the children's beds were in a sorry state. The beddings consisted of dirty old tatters. The ward was literally overflowing with very sick babies, many of them sharing beds. I found some of the children with clinical features I had never seen before when I was a medical student, and later as an intern in mid 1970's in the same ward. There were many emaciated shrivelled children with redundant skin hanging as if unattached to the underlying tissues on spidery limbs, just like loose-fitting gloves. Curiously, for a ward full of children, it was unusually quiet. Evidently most were just too sick to even cry. The silence was obviously a bad omen, as the doomed children seemed to be mourning their own impending deaths.The death rate was very high. I recall the silence being interrupted by intermittent wailings of mothers and relatives in chorus from different parts of the ward following the deaths of their children. Many of the mothers and some of the hospital staff did not look healthy themselves. The spectre of death was all around!

One day, one of my colleagues decided to find out the magnitude of the AIDS problem on our ward by carrying out anonymous HIV tests on all the children. To my horror he reportedly found that almost all the children were HIV positive. The doctor never wanted to talk about it. I just gathered the information from the staff grapevine. This was a turning point for me. There and then I realised that it was AIDS killing almost all my patients. It was therefore the enemy that I had to fight. To be honest, however, I had absolutely no inkling as to how to go about it. I only had the will - but to do what?

Back to the Ward 1C sewage episode: I found out a short time later why it was rather too easy for me to get it fixed. I had wondered why no one else had ever thought of just walking the short distance to the friendly estates officer and asking him to arrange to have it fixed. Somehow I never got a satisfactory answer. That was until one day, a few weeks later, when I narrated the story to a group of friends. One of them was apparently not amused. He suddenly sprang up and rudely interjected: "Gotcha! So you are the villain who caused all that mess?", he exclaimed as he wagged his finger accusingly.

"What mess?" Up until then, I had thought I had cleaned it all up. It transpired that the estates workers asked to repair the sewage channels had simply opened the manhole on the slope just below the hospital. Sewage had flooded the area below the hospital, before overflowing into Gayaza Road which runs parallel to it, making it almost impassable. Following my alarmed report back to estates, it took a bit of emergency civil engineering to reopen the decade long clogged sewage pipes below the road and clean up the unsightly foul-smelling mess. The silver lining, however, was that Ward IC was never flooded again all the time that I worked there. When I visited the ward more recently in 2005 I was pleasantly surprised to find that it had been turned into a clean and nicely maintained cardiac ward.

Facing up to the new threat

On swearing in as the new leader on January 27, 1986, President Museveni promised a fundamental change for a better Uganda. He had fought a protracted bush war to liberate Ugandans from tyranny, suffering and wanton deaths, yet when the break was presented in the form of a hard-won victory, a new and much more treacherous mass killer beyond the reach of military might was annihilating the population. He was to lose to AIDS many more of his brave soldiers than he lost in the entire guerrilla war, over and above the thousands of civilians who also perished. However, President Museveni's leadership with regard to AIDS was a timely blessing, though initially he did not discern the seriousness of the threat, until President Castro of

Cuba started sending back Ugandan trainee soldiers who tested HIV positive.

Museveni demonstrated exceptional foresight and leadership with regard to the crisis, without which many more Ugandans would have died. He was able to do this through a simple but highly practical strategy. First he chose a policy of openness about the disease, thus creating a favourable atmosphere for mass information, education and communication (IEC). At almost all rallies Museveni addressed, he always included a stern warning about AIDS. To the uninfected he talked about prevention in vivid and imaginative terms, aimed at inducing behavioural change. Among other things, he compared irresponsible sex to cows' mating. "As rational humans", Museveni repeatedly emphasised, "people have to be disciplined sexually by sticking to one partner, and not be like cows, in order to avoid AIDS". This was later dubbed "Zero Grazing", using a vivid example of the then newly introduced farming method of rearing cattle in a confined area. Zero grazing cows do not wander around, or get the opportunity to meet with many bulls. These ordinary examples that everyone could relate to captured people's imaginations and set many of them talking and joking about it. If they only joked lightly about this serious problem, there was the menacing sound of the drums on the radio just before and after every news programme to rudely bring them to their senses by warning of the grim threat. Radio ads always started with the beating of the traditional alarm drums warning of impending danger, immediately followed by a sombre booming voice:

BEWARE OF A LOOMING DANGER OF THE KILLER DISEASE -AIDS!
Those who heard it never forgot it. It made hearts thump in peoples' chests. It brought out a cold sweat. Years later, many people, were to openly acknowledge that they would probably be dead if they had not been frightened out of their risky behaviour by this scary advert. Many talked about the chills and shiver the drums used to send down their spines. The net effect was to keep AIDS prevention issues topical,

and the resultant uninhibited talk went a long way towards reducing the stigma and spreading the message. Sensibly, Museveni did not censure the huge numbers already infected or accuse them directly of any wrongdoing. Instead, he urged them to remain responsible citizens, by not spreading the disease, and encouraged them to live positively in hope, while a remedy was being vigorously sought.

Meanwhile, other innovative methods of communicating to the public were initiated and continuously improved upon. Innovative billboards and posters sprang up in all parts of the city and major highways, warning about AIDS, promoting prevention including the use of condoms. When the condom billboards first came out some religious leaders objected, but in time the majority accepted them because of the devastation of AIDS, which their passionate sermons alone could not stop. The first AIDS information and testing centre, funded by United States Agency for International Development (USAID), was opened in central Kampala, and later services were extended upcountry. The initiatives which Museveni inspired, and the interventions that sprang up because of a conducive and open atmosphere, were later to turn around the ravaging epidemic in Uganda. This line of attack needed neither foreign aid nor sophisticated technology. It was just a visionary and timely policy that paid dividends. Taking the cue, the Ministry of Health established the AIDS control programme initially headed by Dr Sam Okware, a hardworking and articulate official who helped in implementing a robust anti-AIDS agenda. Later he was joined by a youthful Dr Warren Namara, who worked hard at promoting AIDS prevention. I was saddened when Warren moved from the Ministry of Health at such a critical time. These two officials were among many others that helped to advance a successful preventive programme for Uganda, which saved many lives. Later the Uganda AIDS Commission (UAC) was initiated by Museveni to mobilise all government ministries in a multi-sectoral partnership to fight the disease. To underscore the importance that the President attached to HIV/AIDS, the new commission was established under the President's office. Uganda's approach became a model, which many countries later emulated.

Countries which kept silent, for various reasons including protection of the tourism industry, or hoping that somehow the disaster would bypass their country, learned to regret it. One good example is that of neighbouring Kenya which remained muted in denial, especially in the 1980's. The government of President Moi initially behaved as if there were no HIV in the country. It was taboo as one courageous Kenyan, Ndinga Achola, found out in 1986. His ordeal started when he declared truthfully that there was AIDS in Kenya. For this utterance alone, he immediately found himself in trouble. Soon after his statement, the police were at his door. He was bundled into a car and taken to a police station for interrogation - read intimidation. Such was the extent of the stigma. When Kenya was finally forced to acknowledge the reality, as was inevitable, a raging epidemic was running riot in their midst.

Although mass information and education about AIDS was critical it was not enough to effectively control the epidemic. Worse still, a very large number of people were already infected and desperately needed at least palliative treatment to ease the suffering. Yet by early 1990's no medicine was available to treat AIDS. It was therefore imperative for Uganda to start a research project to find a cure. However, clinical research, even at the best of times, remains a highly expensive undertaking; yet Uganda, besides being poor, had just emerged from civil wars and a period of anarchy and political upheaval. The country was therefore most ill equipped to deal with the mega catastrophe that AIDS had burdened it with. The situation was made worse by the loss of many productive citizens so desperately needed for leadership in the battered country's recovery. Worse still, the infrastructure was so devastated that it was virtually impossible to find enough funds for the quick rehabilitation of big institutions - - like Uganda's main teaching and referral Mulago Hospital - - to undertake the urgent task of alleviation of the national tragedy. A practical interim move was to start with a small, manageable AIDS research centre, which would be easier to fund. The establishment of the Joint Clinical Research Centre (JCRC) in 1991 was one of Museveni's brilliant ideas aimed at finding a scientific solution. He delegated the important duty to his proficient Chief of Medical Services in the Ugandan military, Dr Ben Mbonye, who headed the new centre for a brief period before I took over. Mbonye helped in the technical planning and establishment of operational principles that have since served the centre well. JCRC was designed to start small, but through prudent policies and hard work it would be expected to grow, find partners and tackle the epidemic scourge. To minimise the cost, the Ugandan military vacated its then operational headquarters to serve as the home of the new centre. This used to be the residence of the Prime Minister *(Katikiro)* of Buganda before 1966 when the Ugandan tribal kingdoms were abolished by the first Obote government. Two other organisations, the Ministry of Health, and Makerere University, were brought on board together with the Ministry of Defence in a strategic partnership to support the efforts of the new centre. The Ministry of Health was to provide policy guidance; Makerere University was to provide scientists and researchers, while the Ministry of Defence catered for infrastructure. The centre was given autonomous status as a non-profit making limited liability company, to avoid bureaucratic impediments, and to mandate it to seek partners and independent funding.

The government provided the JCRC with some basic laboratory equipment to start it off. This included the then state-of-the-art flowcytometer machine, the very first in East and Central Africa, to measure CD4 cells. Other essential but simpler laboratory equipment were borrowed from Mbuya Military Hospital, so that scientific research on anti-AIDS products, both herbal and formal drugs, which could possibly alleviate the desperate plight of Ugandans, could start right away. At that time when the sophistication of the HIV pathogenesis was poorly understood, it was widely believed that an AIDS cure could be easily discovered. In fact, the research agenda seemed to work almost immediately. By early 1992, two important drugs trials were underway at the JCRC. They included the very first antiretroviral trial in Africa involving the only approved AIDS drug of the time, Zidovudine, better known as AZT. This was undertaken in partnership with the University of California San Francisco (UCSF). Burroughs Wellcome, the AZT manufacturer, funded the study. At the time AZT used to be prescribed in high doses in an effort to obtain superior treatment outcome.

Unfortunately this was associated with nasty toxic effects, some of them fatal. JCRC was one of the pioneer institutions to demonstrate that AZT was just as effective when used with low doses, but with the added advantage of a much better safety profile. Unfortunately, commercial interests in AZT and other emerging antiretroviral (ARV) drugs denied the JCRC follow-up research opportunities. It was to take almost ten years before other major antiretroviral pharmaceutical companies would support another study involving U.S. approved ARV drugs in Uganda.

Despite the humble beginning, and meagre funds, the role of the JCRC - - which was, as it were, started expressly to urgently fight the AIDS scourge - - was to grow. Its influence extended beyond the borders of Uganda, inspired, galvanised and helped revolutionise access to care and treatment throughout the resource-constrained countries of the world. However, to get to this stage, there were immense compounding factors which I as the centre's head encountered. Just as the situation looked irredeemably gloomy, some totally unexpected events emerged that were to radically change the whole AIDS scenario of doom and despair to one of cautious optimism.

However, before going deeper into some aspects of my long, eventful and intricate involvement in the struggle against AIDS, I need to take the reader back in time to the beginning of AIDS in Uganda - - the very first epicentre of the epidemic in Africa. And throw some light on some of the reasons that I think made it such a devastating disaster.

Chaos and melodrama

Idi Amin's January 1971 coup d'état found me at Makerere University, Kampala, where I studied medicine up to my graduation in 1975. The 1970s were very difficult times for Ugandans. Idi Amin's regime was busy tearing down the country, terrorising the citizenry and neighbouring countries alike, while at the same time mesmerizing the world with the most incredible gimmicks. Yet the connection with what was to unfold out of it all would leave the best of fortune-tellers totally mystified! In fact, the only sexually transmitted disease that Amin was worried about at the time was gonorrhoea; and accordingly, tongue in cheek, he issued a warning to Makerere University students about the danger. Actually, he accused the students of spreading the terrible disease. Little did Amin (or indeed anyone else for that matter) know that right at that very time a much more vicious scourge, which would make gonorrhoea look like a common cold was incubating in Uganda.

In hindsight, it is amazing how some seemingly unrelated political and bad governance issues combined with the resultant social economic consequences would bounce back to haunt and devastate a nation. A few glimpses of Amin's regime's excesses, the bizarre events and the resultant state of affairs paints a picture of what was going on while HIV was insidiously burgeoning in the country. But it was not always apparent how such events played a role in both incubating and effectively shielding HIV from earlier detection in Uganda. However, there is no doubt that the 1970s chaos fuelled it in one way or the other. What remains unclear is merely the magnitude.

In fact, if Amin had stayed on a little longer, I am of the view that Africa would have most likely been "honoured" with her third emperor. There was just no other direction to a higher and glorious ground left for him to take. In the meantime, Amin just had to contend with the topmost but comparatively ordinary rank of Field Marshal and the comparatively less prestigious office of Life President of Uganda. But the creative Marshal then made up some special titles for himself, including "Conqueror of British Empire--CBE" and also awarded himself the top British war heroes' award; "The Victorian Cross --VC". To go with all his self-imposed titles, Amin had to buy impressive military hardware including Soviet Supersonic Mig Fighters, tanks and artillery in addition to the vehicles and other equipment to match his status. Finally he had to provoke a war to demonstrate his invincibility. In preparation, the Field Marshal expanded the army by importing royal Nubian mercenaries from South Sudan to protect him, exterminate his enemies and carry out his whims. Ugandans loathed and despised the cruel mercenaries whose tribal tattoos in the form of stripes on either side of their rugged cheeks dubbed *"one hundred and eleven"*, betrayed their identity. However, all these were very expensive undertakings, yet Uganda's production and exports were at an all time low.

In another erratic operation that he dubbed "Economic War", on August 4, 1972, Amin recklessly expelled about 60,000 Asian businessmen and their families who were the backbone of the Ugandan economy, giving them 90 days to leave the country. The Asians, mainly of Indian origin, dominated the running of factories, commerce and other economically important sectors partly because of the relatively favoured positions they held over indigenous Africans during colonial times. Therefore this move was quite popular with many Ugandans because they viewed Asians as a highly privileged and sectarian group. Amin on his side accused them of "milking the cow without feeding it." However, after they were gone Amin just killed the cow.

The Asians' abrupt forced departure left a vacuum in the business sector that Amin rapidly filled with greenhorns -- with disastrous consequences. He did it as part reward and part bribe to his cronies, most of whom had absolutely no trade experience. All that most of them did was to sell the stock found in the shops at any price, without re-stocking simply because they had no idea it was necessary. Ugandans watched with utter disbelief, as some shops previously stocked with trendy jewellery, hi-fi and television sets transformed into selling bananas. The net effect of this fiasco was to greatly impoverish Ugandans, as the already weakened economy collapsed. The shattering effect it had on the population was believed by many to have played a role in creating an enabling environment for AIDS to thrive partly by increased sex for favours and money. In addition, economic hardships and other resultant adverse factors combined to synthesize such chaotic conditions that veiled early recognition of the emerging epidemic.

The real commerce in town was hijacked by a streetwise new generation of peddlers, petty traders and smugglers who came to be known as *bayaye*. The *bayaye* developed their own underground lingua franca and jargon dubbed "Luyaye," in which they communicated to escape the vicious anti-smuggling squad. In addition, on January, 8 1975, Amin declared that overcharging, hoarding of scarce goods, and cheating were treasonable offences punishable by death. The dreaded squad ostensibly set up to counter such illegal activities were in reality the godfathers of *bayaye*. Marshal Idi Amin, who was barely literate, and his Vice-President General Mustafa Idris, who was totally illiterate, did not have any inkling or evident concerns about the country's economy, which they ran like a medieval chieftain's empire. The Kampala rumour mill had it that the very first time General Mustafa heard about the difficulties Ugandans were experiencing with regard to the foreign exchange, his first thought was that "Foreign Exchange" was the leader of a new insurgency that needed to be eliminated. The grapevine chat had it that the fearless general reacted immediately to the threat by cocking his Kalashnikov, announcing that he was ready to defend the country by gunning down the felonious "Mr Foreign Exchange," "Mr F.E," as the grapevine called it. Years later, long after the fall of his boss Amin, Mustafa appeared before the human rights commission of inquiry where he was specifically asked to explain what quarrel he had with Mr FE. The General pleaded "innocent" insisting that he really bore no grudge against him. He further shocked the commission when he admitted that as Vice-President of Uganda, he could neither read nor understand any of the official documents. As for the constitution, he just had no idea that it existed.

On the other hand, Amin had a more practical solution than his deputy Mustafa to the critical problem of shortage of the money needed to buy his military toys and to keep his henchmen happy. He just printed more money. Inescapably, inflation skyrocketed as the country went from inflation to hyper-inflation, reaching an incredible 1,000 %. Civil servants' salaries became almost worthless. As a newly qualified doctor my monthly salary was just enough to purchase half a basket of mangoes!

However, Amin had a rather soft spot for us doctors. In 1975, as intern doctors, we rather naively went on strike, perhaps the only serious one in his entire reign. Our strike was viewed so seriously that Amin personally had to make the short three-kilometre journey from his camp in Kololo, a suburb of Kampala, to Mulago teaching hospital to address us. Everyone of us feared that the unpredictable general would order our immediate arrest, torture and possibly execution. To a man whose regime later murdered the country's Chief Justice, an Archbishop, senior ministers, diplomats, academicians (including the vice-chancellor of the then country's only university), bankers, down to peasant villagers, mere junior doctors would not be an issue. To make matters worse for us, the then dean of the medical school, abandoned us to our fate and condemned our strike, informing Idi Amin that as interns we were not real doctors. Worse still, the then civilian Minister of Health did not spare a kind word in our favour, but condemned our strike as totally unjustified and intolerable. In retrospect, this was unbelievable, considering that our lives were in mortal danger. It appears to me that these two officials were over enthusiastically trying to impress Amin and be recorded in his good books. If this was their intention, they failed. They were both to flee for dear life into exile where they lived until after Amin was overthrown.

Any form of rebellion against Amin was always ruthlessly punished. His preferred method of operation against perceived opponents, even if they were falsely accused, as was often the case, was to hit them hard (read, kill them dead) before they sprang. On January, 24 and February, 12 1973, there were shocking countrywide public executions by firing squad of people, each one in his hometown, who were alleged to have conspired against Amin. This is the context in which our rather foolhardy strike may be viewed. However, with our youthful exuberance and invincibility, we were not fully aware and certainly not prepared for any ghastly eventuality, though initially we postured to feed and impress our over inflated egos and each other. Yet all that we wanted and could probably have died for was a mere salary rise from Shillings 1200 to Shillings 1800, per month, now equivalent to less than one US dollar. Just that! The public salary review committee set up by Amin himself had in fact recommended the increase but this had not been implemented, and thus our strike. This was the background to our predicament as we came face to face with the formidable Idi Amin himself in person. There we were in Davis Lecture Theatre of Makerere Medical School, like cats on a hot tin roof, taking some comfort in our numbers, listening with disbelief as our bosses condemned us to our fate. You could have heard a pin drop!

However, our downcast sprits were on the spur of the moment lifted up when Amin started his speech by addressing us as "My fellow doctors." We cheered the dictator as we saw some ray of hope in his opening remark. What a welcome relief it was. The Field Marshal's magical three words offered us some hope. Though the tension eased a bit, we still realised with trepidation that we were not yet out of the woods. Amin was not known to forget or forgive any dissent, however minor. Therefore we still fearfully awaited the punishment that he would dish out. Amin was also not known to give light punishments. We knew very well that whomever Amin punished, remained punished. So, we waited fearfully, holding on with baited breath, clinging only to the shared title, hoping against hope that Amin somehow and somewhere in his inner heart reserved some special consideration for his "colleagues". The shared title of "doctor" was in reference to an honorary Doctor of Laws degree that was conferred upon him by Makerere University under duress. From then onwards he had to be addressed as "Doctor" without fail among many other titles that he had awarded himself. To our profound relief, Amin did not seem to view the strike as seriously as the minister and the dean did. He talked a lot of good things that he wished to do for his fellow "doctors". He had absolutely no hesitation in granting us the demanded salary rise, as he pushed aside the protestation of the minister. Oh, how I wished we had asked for more!

Amin went further and authorised "his colleagues" the "dactars" to be given special vouchers to access essential supplies at subsidised prices from the highly restricted government Foods and Beverages Stores. This was normally a special privilege reserved for the select or favoured few. That was the only way to make our joke of a salary pay for anything. However, there was a catch. When we excitedly went to partake of our newly conferred privilege, we found to our consternation that there were in fact two entrances and different times for entering the store, which was often empty by the times we were granted access. There was absolutely no need to bother with the making of a shopping list, as there was no way to tell what would be found in stock. Thus someone else within the store always took the decision of what one would purchase. In 1976, I remember lining up for hours, but when I finally entered there were only tinned green peas left. As even these were not enough to go round, I was rationed to buy only two small tins. As fate would have it, I arrived home with only one. A friend's wife, who had earlier offered me a lift, stole the other. This was very understandable and readily pardonable as many people had so little to eat that tinned peas would be considered a delicacy. Many were living on the verge of starvation. It was his cronies, especially those that bumped off his enemies and terrorised the people that had priority access. They were the same ones that cruised menacingly around town in the latest models of Fiat and Peugeot cars as they frolicked with the best girls in town - - or just married them often forcefully and not infrequently after murdering their rivals. Upcountry in the villages where the majority of Ugandans lived, the situation was even worse. The villagers in rural areas lacked even the very basic supplies like salt, sugar and soap. My father once told me about an old woman who turned up in the small southern town of Rukungiri with a pumpkin for sale. Asked about the price, the old lady responded, "I want a million shilling!" to the bemusement of the vendors, and went on to explain her reasons for the price tag. "I hear that's what you pay for everything these days." Although the old lady did not get her million shillings, she still walked home with enough money that in terms of figures would have fetched her a brand new saloon car only six years before. However, in terms of the then value the large bundle of paper money that she laboriously took home was just enough for a candy.

Amin had also choked up the country's other lifelines for foreign aid, which could have made the lives of Ugandans a little better. He did it by his astounding blunders and buffoonery that incensed the donors, leaving those he did not expel with no other option but to close shop and quit. On March, 23 1972, Amin gave the Israelis only four days to leave Uganda. Following the expulsion of the marines who guarded the embassy in Kampala, the USA closed her embassy and quit Uganda in November, 1973. The British, on the other hand, lingered on a little longer. However, by mid 1976, they were thoroughly fed up with Amin, and on July, 4 broke off diplomatic relations with Uganda, leaving the French as caretakers of their dwindling interests in the country. Thus Uganda became increasingly isolated as more countries closed their embassies. Never mind that some of these countries, especially Britain and Israel, were buoyed up by Idi Amin's coup d'état. The West initially turned a blind eye to the bloody aftermath, and in the beginning supported him morally and materially. This was mainly because his predecessor, Mr Apollo Obote, who, incidentally, also insisted on being called "Doctor" for the same reasons as Amin, was perceived as a communist crony because of his leftist leanings. Some people still believe that without clandestine support from Israel and Britain, Amin's coup would not have succeeded. Jimmy Carter was later to say of Amin's policies that they "disgusted the entire civilised world", but before that Amin had his back against the Western leaders who shunned him.

Starting with the beleaguered President Nixon, then in the midst of the Watergate scandal that was to lead to his impeachment, Amin wrote, tongue in cheek, to wish him "a quick recovery from Watergate." Turning to Her Majesty, the Queen of the United Kingdom, he offered Ugandan cabbages and bananas "to save the starving Britons." He followed up the generous offer by calling upon Ugandans to donate charitably. Yet charity begins at home, and many more Ugandans than Britons did not have enough for themselves. Therefore, Amin sent his scouts to obtain the food donation under coercion. He then invited the press to assemble at the collection points to witness the historical event. However, the press was not invited to cover the actual shipment because it was never meant to happen. The "donated" foodstuffs, some of which were already at Entebbe airport, were distributed to his friends and henchmen while the country was facing food shortages.

When even this show failed to impress the British, Amin plotted to bring them to their knees. He arrested a Briton by the name of Denis Hills, a teacher living in Uganda. Amin's secret agents caught Mr Hills writing a book entitled *The White Pumpkin* in which he described Amin as a "black Nero" and a "village tyrant". In revenge, Amin threatened to execute him despite numerous desperate appeals for clemency, including that of Her Majesty the Queen of United Kingdom. Amin demanded a top-level apology and the then British Prime Minister Harold Wilson wrote one. But it was all to no avail. Increasing the stakes, Amin demanded that the British should go down on their knees to beg him to spare Hill's life. Of course, no self-respecting British official was prepared to voluntarily kneel at Idi Amin's feet. But the nifty Amin had his own uncanny ways of ensuring that his wishes always came true. When the Queen sent her envoy General Blair to negotiate Hills' release, Amin arranged for the meeting to take place in the remote north-western Ugandan rural village of Koboko. There he had a modified traditional hut specially constructed for the momentous reception. When the British General arrived in Uganda swearing that he would not kneel to Amin, he soon found out that he had to do exactly that. The envoy was told that the meeting would take place in the hut that Amin had specially designed with a long low entrance. The Queen's envoy On Her Majesty's Service carrying an official appeal for clemency to Amin had to crawl on all fours through the low, dark narrow entrance. As he emerged in the well lit interior the cameras were busy snapping away as the beaming dictator sat on a chief's chair savouring the sight of a full British general kneeling at his feet. Yet even this self-indulgence was not enough for Amin to secure Hills' release. The British general went back empty-handed as Amin hurled insults at him on top of trumped up accusations that he had partaken of too much *Uganda Waragi*, a potent local gin. Overnight *Uganda Waragi* was temporarily renamed "General Blair" by the highly impressionable Ugandan bar-goers in all Kampala's pubs and drinking joints. To encourage the British to act expeditiously on his threats, Amin made it look like the execution was imminent. Promptly the British government hurriedly sent their Foreign Secretary, James Callaghan (who was later to become the British Prime Minister and then Lord Callaghan), to save Hills. Weary of Amin's monkey tricks, Callaghan hatched a plot using a secret weapon, which he disclosed to the British Parliament two decades later on Tuesday December, 16 1997, as follows:

I think there are illustrations and if I say to you, as I do, that I actually used Mobutu, that man, in order to assist in the release of Dennis Hills, was I right or was I wrong? I have no doubt about the answer to that, but it so happened that Amin owed certain debts to Mobutu, not just in money but in other ways, and so when I went to rescue Dennis Hills, I went first to Zaire and breakfasted off a gold plate in his penthouse suite, with the lions roaring below, and got him to send with me to Uganda his Foreign Secretary, and his Foreign Secretary saw Amin before I saw Amin, and we worked it all out between us. Now, here was an example of using a dictator of the worst possible kind in order to do a deal with another dictator that you thought would do some good. Now, here are the dilemmas. It is all very well for the theoretical practitioners to talk about these matters, but these are the dilemmas that you have to think of.

Unlike the over 300,000 Ugandans and a score of foreigners who were brutally murdered and millions who suffered torture, untold hardship and terror, on June 10, 1976, Hills was released by Amin and whisked away by Callaghan narrowly escaping with his life. He lived to the ripe age of 90.

But Amin was not yet finished with the British. He had one more trick up his sleeve. In one notorious basement in Nakasero, an upper class suburb of Kampala, was the "slaughter chamber in section C2" where the vicious so called State Research (the death squad) murdered thousands of Amin's real, framed or imagined enemies. Most of the victims were there on false charges or for trivial reasons like business or love rivalries. In 1977, a group of brutally tortured prisoners being held there on verge of death were surprised by a sudden change in treatment. They were told that this unexpected lull in their daily vicious torture sessions, or "cups of tea" (as the torturers, led by the sadist one Minawa, called them in their jargon), was because Amin was in a forgiving mood while he pondered their possible release as a goodwill gesture towards the British. This was yet another of Amin's disingenuous tactics of inveigling his way into the limelight ahead of the prestigious Commonwealth Heads of Governments meeting (CHOGM) that was scheduled to take place in Britain towards the end of 1977. However, Britain had made it clear that the "monstrous" Idi Amin would not be welcome. Defiantly, the mischievous Marshal Amin threatened to gatecrash the meeting. True to his word, the life President announced to the hastily called press conference that he was on his way to London. Thus he had all the startled British and some European radar systems operators working overtime scanning the skies on the lookout for the dictator's plane. The world's news media scrambled to take positions at various airports along the expected route to scoop an exclusive breaking news story of Amin's historic landing and the unpredictable repercussions or drama that would unfold. Meanwhile, Royal Air Force planes remained on full alert ready to intercept his plane on sight. In the meantime, rumour in Kampala had it that the impish tyrant just landed his presidential Gulf Stream jet at the Ugandan Air force base of Nakasongora, about 100 km north of Kampala, parked it in a Ugandan Air force shed, and then just returned to town by road. Other grapevine talk had it that he just paid a surprise visit to his friend President Gadaffi in Tripoli, Libya, and then returned. In reality he never left Kampala. Anyway, by the time his plane was expected in European air space, Idi was said to be comfortably ensconced in his reclining chair relaxing in his backyard, his legs up, orange juice by his side, tuned to the BBC with an interpreter explaining the "difficult" words, gleefully enjoying the drama in Europe as it unfolded.

Only rarely was any of Amin's tomfoolery in good taste. For instance, to the elderly lady Israel Prime Minister, Golda Meir, Amin wrote an open letter about her "knickers!" "Arab victory in the war with Israel is inevitable and prime minister of Israel Mrs Golda Meir's only recourse is to tuck up her knickers and run away in the direction of New York and Washington," the infamous letter read in part. Yet this was in no way the worst of his outrages against the Israelis who had cheered and, some say, engineered his ascendancy to power. When the Israeli commandoes raided Entebbe airport to rescue their citizens hijacked by the Palestinians and held with the help of Amin on July 3, 1976, one elderly Israeli woman, Dora Block, who had earlier been taken ill in Mulago hospital was brutally murdered in revenge. Her name and the words, "DORA BLOCK WAS HERE" were found scribbled on the wall of the torture and murder chamber C1, in Nakasero, according to one Mr Apollo Lawoko, a Ugandan survivor who wrote a heart-wrenching, harrowing account of the torture and deaths that he witnessed there.

Even Amin's neighbours were not spared. On November, 5,1978, Amin the former local boxing champion, wrote to the aging neighbouring President of Tanzania, Julius Nyerere, challenging him to a boxing match. In a double outrage, he mockingly offered to have his right hand tied tightly behind his back during the duel. Then in a dramatic turnaround, the erratic dictator declared his unconditional "love" for Nyerere. "I love you so much that I would marry you if you were a woman!" his letter read. However, instead of expressing his true love by sending flowers, Amin instead sent his forces to invade Nyerere's Tanzania.

In this truly Ugandan tragedy of the 1970's, the country was hardly ever out of the news - - and for the wrong reasons, including the wacky episodes described above. The world's comedians and publishers of comic magazines, including *Punch* of London, had a field day acting out and publishing Amin's devices that kept the world transfixed and tied in knots in amusement. But to the hapless Ugandans under the dictator's iron grip, the dire circumstances were not funny. The people suffered tremendously both physically, and psychologically, as chaos prevailed. Virtually everything disappeared from the shops - - and anything that could somehow be found was just unaffordable. Henry Kyemba, one of the first of Amin's ministers who later fled the mayhem, published a book about Amin's atrocities, appropriately entitled *The State of Blood* In it he described shocking carnage and the chaotic situation. Any Ugandan lucky enough to get hold of the bits and pieces of essential goods, like table salt or bathing soap, would often find themselves in serious trouble. They could be accused of smuggling, a crime that could carry a death sentence carried out in the most gruesome ways. Amin-style executions included use of hammers or bayonets. In its most brutal version, a badly tortured prisoner would be promised life if he hammered another one to death. What the hapless fellow did not realise was that as soon as he has finished the heinous act, he would then be the very next in line for slaughter. This gruesome exercise would go on until the very last one remained. However, his life expectancy would be counted in hours rather than days. The most gruesome torture in Uganda took place mainly in the upper chamber of the notorious so-called "State Research" or human "butchery" at Nakasero. In such brutal circumstances, human respect was at its lowest ebb, self-esteem minimal, and the moral fabric of society broken as people struggled to survive, and sex for favours increased. Indeed the country was going through many fast moving events, which the then strongman at the helm, Marshal Idi Amin, once described as moving at a "supersonic speed." This was quite right, but Amin had engaged the reverse gear.

The rescue of Ugandans from Amin's reign of terror came rather unexpectedly towards the end of 1978. This followed a botched-up invasion of the Tanzanian Kagera river basin on September 9 by Amin's soldiers claiming that it was a part of Uganda. The following day Amin's Soviet-made and equipped air force bombed Tanzania. Meanwhile the undisciplined army on ground killed, raped and indiscriminately looted extensively. As the Tanzanians retaliated, Amin fled from Mutukula on the Uganda's southern border with Tanzania, all the way across the country to Sudan, with the Tanzanian People's Defence Force and a rag-tag Ugandan exile force right on his heels.

During the entire Amin regime (1970 – 1979) an estimated 300,000 to 400,000 Ugandans were murdered, and many others, especially the much-needed elite, fled into exile. As Amin, who was on several occasions accused of shameful cowardice by his peers (including one Brigadier Okoya who did not live long after making the accusation), took to his heels, he left behind a people in abject poverty. Amin fled into exile first in Libya, and on to Saudi Arabia where he later died, without facing the law to answer for the many atrocities attributed to him in Uganda and abroad. He left behind a country in ruins, as well as social, cultural and economic turmoil from which it has never fully recovered.

He also left behind a burgeoning disease that in terms of the carnage was to make the massacre of his regime fade into oblivion by comparison.

The Birth of AIDS

Following Amin's ousting on April, 11 1979, the whole country exploded into lengthy celebrations interspersed with widespread looting in Kampala. Roadside comedians acted out humorous dramatic plays based on vivid imaginings and graphic interpretations of Amin's humiliating defeat and cowardly retreat. The spectre of the invincible general huffing and puffing in full retreat captured many people's imaginations. Naturally, the relief was much more pronounced among those who had suffered directly under his cruel regime. Some went as far as improvising effigies of the fallen "Field Marshal" and venting their decade-long anger and frustrations on the hapless dummies. Many aggrieved folks never imagined that in their lifetime they would witness the brutal dictator on the receiving end.

The festivities however, died out rather too prematurely in Rakai, as the startled residents there increasingly realised that while one nightmare was ending another one - creepy and very mysterious - was unfolding in their midst. Most perturbing of all, whereas Amin's totalitarian regime was at times indiscriminate in massacring the citizens, the new curse seemed to select the young and the well-off at their peak. It looked like a gruesome decapitation of the next generation. The new scourge in Uganda emerged from the ashes of Idi Amin's era. It was born into the new post-Amin political turmoil and wars of the early 1980's that provided a fertile ground to thrive insidiously; initially but later to overtake California, thus making Uganda the undisputed world's epicentre of the pandemic.

It now seems inevitable to link the relentless spread of AIDS in Uganda with the reign of terror that perpetuated insurgency and impoverished the population, resulting in the breakdown of traditional family and community ways of life. The cultural norms that regulated sexual behaviour were to a considerable extent disrupted as the country degenerated into anarchy and economic collapse. Amin's marauding forces were suspected by some of being responsible for the early spread of HIV in 1970s. However, it seems that their main contribution to the introduction of AIDS in Uganda was through the chaos that they perpetuated - which created conducive conditions for its establishment, and the hardships that promoted the risky behaviour that fuelled it. Although Amin's soldiers were not prominent among the very early casualties of AIDS, by the end of the bush war in 1986, the Ugandan soldiers who replaced them, and especially the guerrilla army, had emerged as a distinct AIDS high-risk group. It is probable that without the chaos, AIDS would not have hit Uganda so early and so much harder than any other country in the world.

At independence in 1962, Uganda was one of the most promising countries in Africa. The country, as the tourist promotion slogan goes, is indeed gifted by nature. It is endowed with considerable natural resources and good weather throughout the year. The transition from colonial Britain was relatively smooth and the new Prime Minister, Milton Obote, though only semi-educated, started off very well with broad national support. He was able to forge alliances with the influential Buganda kingdom, and other Ugandan multi-tribal constituencies, promising a bright future for the new country. Unfortunately ideological divisions, intrigue and inter-sectarian conflicts crept in and were allowed by the short-sighted regime to thrive in order to consolidate political and military power. Only three and half years later, on May, 24 1966, the army led by Amin, on Obote's orders attacked the Buganda king's palace and ousted him, thus precipitating a crisis that culminated in the abolition of the constitutional tribal kingdoms on September, 17 1967. As a prelude, five independent minded government ministers accused of plotting against Obote were arrested at a fake cabinet meeting in February 1966, amidst increasing intolerance and dissent. This cleared the way for Obote to overthrow the country's constitution and impose a new one dubbed the "pigeon hole constitution" on April, 15 1966. This was so called because many members of parliament voted for it with hardly any inkling about the contents, as the draft had been put in their pigeon holes the very night before the crucial vote. They soon found out, however, that the new constitution had transformed Prime Minister Obote into the executive President of Uganda with sweeping powers. This formed the background to the subsequent turmoil and mayhem. Moving from the frying pan into the fire, Idi Amin deposed Obote on January 25, 1971, and within a short time became a much worse tyrant. Almost a decade later, when a combined force of Tanzanian and Ugandan exile forces put an end to Amin's reign of terror, the situation had got much worse. Incidentally, the invading Tanzanian forces were also suspected by the Rakai villagers of playing a role in the introduction and spread of HIV in the area. However, considering that clinical AIDS has a long incubation period, this seems highly unlikely as the Tanzanians army first passed through Rakai too close to the emergence of the first cases of full-blown AIDS in the area.

It was not until September 1982 that the first cases of advanced AIDS were clearly documented by Dr Nelson Sewankambo and his colleagues in Uganda. However, as we now know that the incubation period of AIDS can take up to ten years and occasionally even beyond, it means that the disease had in fact been spreading during the disarray of the 1970s. Residents of Rakai and the neighbouring Tanzania area had earlier on noted what Dr Sewankambo and his colleagues later documented. The wars, resultant chaos, and Amin's gaffes that had held the world spell-bound in amazement while Uganda faced economic collapse and hardships had concealed an AIDS time bomb. When it exploded in the early 1980s it triggered off a devastating nationwide epidemic that was to wreak havoc on the population.

Regarding political leadership, hapless Ugandans did not enjoy a much-deserved respite after Amin's brutal regime. His overthrow was followed in quick succession by five short-lived regimes and non-stop pandemonium that ended after 1986, by which time AIDS was fully established as a catastrophic epidemic in the country. Incredibly, among the five mainly autocratic post-Amin leaders, was the same Obote whom Amin ousted in 1979. Given or rather grabbing a second chance, Obote, renowned for his love of the bottle, not surprisingly repeated the same blunders complete with the appointment of yet another illiterate despot soldier Tito Okello as the army boss. Tito in turn kicked him out just as Amin had done. Obote's human rights record and the number of people killed during his second regime rivalled Amin's. Indeed, the legacy of Obote's second regime includes the massacres that took place in the central region, known as "the Luwero triangle". There, thousands of human skulls, akin to a mini-version of the Rwandan genocide aftermath, were discovered after he was overthrown from power by his illiterate army commander General Tito Okello Lutwa. The gruesome skulls were for a while displayed as a shocking reminder of the pain Ugandans suffered under Obote's reign (1981-1986).

Mercifully for poor Uganda, Okello's rowdy regime after Obote was short lived, as he too fled Amin-style the onslaught of a much more disciplined force led by an idealistic guerrilla fighter, Yoweri Museveni, in 1986. However, by that time the AIDS scourge was so serious that one prominent expatriate surgeon, Dr Carswell, underscored the seriousness of the matter by implying that the Ugandan population was on the verge of being decimated. "Come back to Uganda in a few years, there will be plenty of parking spaces in Kampala," the doctor was reported to have said. The remark earned him the unfortunate title of "persona non grata" as he was unceremoniously deported from Uganda back to his native Scotland in April 1987.

I remember feeling disappointed by the news of his deportation, as I personally knew the beleaguered surgeon as a good, down-to-earth, kind man and a great humanitarian. I worked under him as an intern doctor and admired his work. He braved the chaotic Ugandan regimes including that of Idi Amin, which was so vicious that almost all other expatriates fled. The skilled surgeon had learnt to improvise his own ways of survival during the harsh times including, as I later gathered, rearing his own pigs in his backyard for food. He was a workaholic, who stayed late in Mulago hospital operating on seriously ill patients including many emergencies with bullet wounds sustained from Amin's trigger-happy thugs. While some of the few Ugandan doctors that did not flee struggled for survival by moonlighting in private clinics, Carswell was always there holding the fort. He could always be relied upon to attend to surgical emergencies and if there were no facilities for the operation, as was often the case, he would come up with amazing improvisations in order to save the patient. He undoubtedly saved many lives and very much deserved a medal instead of deportation. There was also some whispering that he was a mole because of his extraordinary resilience during the brutal period of Amin's reign, but the simple life that he led in Uganda and continued to live in Britain after his deportation don't bear this out. He was, as far as I could judge, just a selfless humanitarian and an innocent victim of the AIDS stigma.

However, the fact that such a man was deported for articulating what was clearly at the back of everyone's mind is a clear indication of how stigmatized and jittery many people, felt about AIDS, including the Ministry of Health authorities. There was so much fear of AIDS that even talking about it brought on the creeps.

The AIDS Time Bomb

Many have tried to figure out how insecurity, terror, chaos, political volatility, wars and economic collapse could have possibly constituted an AIDS time bomb in Uganda, and later in other parts of Africa. Many still wonder what the exact connection, was with, for instance, the events that unfolded in Uganda under Idi Amin. Some, perhaps too hastily, thought they could read a clear cut link. However, this may have been just a rash oversimplification, as the evidence remains indistinct. It is perhaps safer in the meantime to presuppose that cause and effect may in such a messy situation only be defined in a roundabout way until better evidence emerges. However, AIDS being the most controversial infectious illness since the Black Death, virtually everyone, novice and professional, feels they have something to say about it -The true picture requires detailed study. Nevertheless, some of the current evidence seems to indicate that AIDS evolvement is a highly complex phenomenon encompassing many facets that are yet to be comprehensively described. Superficial interpretations and assumptions have in the past raised many more questions than answers. Many current theories and publications on the subject produce conflicting results.

Undeniably the earliest cases of AIDS in Africa were documented in Uganda. But almost certainly it did not originate there. Nevertheless, Uganda has variously been described as AIDS ground zero – By the early 1990s, the AIDS epidemic had peaked in Uganda. The country was then the world's unchallenged AIDS epicentre in terms of infection rates and deaths. However, this was only until the mid 1990s when the epicentre shifted decisively and more destructively southwards. Therefore it is imperative that events that preceded or existed during the AIDS flare-up in Uganda, even if they might initially appear unrelated, be carefully examined and dissected for any possible clue to the origin, spread and devastation brought by AIDS to the country. However, political upheaval, bad leadership and other kinds of chaos, especially in conflict-riddled Africa, were not a sole monopoly of Uganda. Therefore events pertaining to the evolution of the epidemic in other parts of the continent and beyond may be compared and contrasted with the Ugandan experience in an effort to throw some light on this complex matter.

Such an opportunity to further examine the possible cause-effect was presented when history seemed to repeat itself but at the same time offered some essential differences. A similar or worse socioeconomic scenario to Uganda's was reproduced two decades later one thousand five hundred air miles south - in Zimbabwe. However, unlike Uganda, the strong man at the helm in Harare, Robert Mugabe, was astute and well educated, and his government was not like Amin and Obote's admittedly. Until the end of 1990s Zimbabwe was the breadbasket - or should we call it the maize meal granary - of southern Africa. Like Uganda, the country had a promising start despite the ravages of the war of independence. The problems started when Mugabe forcefully evicted many white farmers, who were the backbone of Zimbabwe's agriculture and economy, to address a gross injustice of the past.

The white farmers under the hard-line racist system had ruthlessly grabbed the land from the poor Africans who desperately depended on it for their very survival. The native African evictees were left without any compensation or any reasonable humanitarian consideration. Land had been what the liberation war had been all about. Understandably, therefore, the injustice needed to be addressed, and even Britain the former colonial power promised to help Zimbabwe. However, Mugabe seemed to lose patience as the promised relief did not materialise. The manner in which Mugabe went about it as well as the repercussions bruised Zimbabwe. The Previously highly productive farms were redistributed to landless indigenous Zimbabweans, but proportionally more to Mugabe's cronies and some ruling party members, who by and large never had a chance during the white segregationist rule to learn anything about farming. This deed turned the relatively well-off Zimbabwe from a net exporter of food into a state with chronic severe food shortages and subsequent hardships for the population. Understandably, Mugabe's actions met with Western countries' wrath resulting in a damaging standoff between the immovable Mugabe and the West led by Britain. In addition, a well orchestrated negative publicity campaign turned Mugabe into a pariah figure.

In response, the increasingly besieged Mugabe, the master orator, launched a hard-hitting verbal counterattack which only served to harden the western countries' determination to dish out harsher punitive measures against him. Some of his utterances, though articulately delivered in impeccable English, were received in the West in the same way as Amin's ramblings. Despite a chorus of protests, Mugabe steadfastly remained defiant (just as Amin did), seemingly oblivious to his country going to the dogs. Mugabe, the veteran guerrilla commander, was not unfamiliar with hardships, having endured worse during the long war of independence. Characteristically he was on the warpath declaring that: "It is preferable to die fighting instead of living as squatters in our own land." In his resolve, Mugabe was encouraged by the fact that the seizures of white-owned farms were very popular with big sections of the community, especially the very poor, just as Amin's expulsion of the Asian business community had been in Uganda. The reaction to Mugabe's action from the West was the same as Amin got: a vindictive rebuff and the imposition of crushing economic sanctions. To top it off they slammed a travel ban on him and his top officials. All this resulted in the economic ruin of his country. Consequently, the country was hit by a devastating runaway inflation that surpassed a staggering 2000 %. In later years it was to climb to unbelievable levels of well over 5000%. Zimbabwe's battered population faced untold destitution as they shovelled around bags of valueless paper money that looked like poor quality monopoly game cards. This was very reminiscent of the bleak Ugandan situation of the 1970s and early 1980s. The increasingly starving population, unable to make ends meet, and facing an increasingly repressive regime took to their heels and fled mainly to South Africa and Botswana as economic refugees.

In this unfolding chaos, AIDS hit Zimbabwe initially insidiously but in time exploded into a devastating scourge that propelled Zimbabwe from one of the lowest HIV affected countries in Africa to become one of the most hard hit countries with one of the highest rates in the world ten years later. Many descriptions of the evolution of AIDS epidemic in Uganda from the 1980s and early 1990s could be lifted from the Uganda narrative above and pasted in the Zimbabwe section here and they would fit almost perfectly. Therefore, in consideration of these almost similar events, it would be logical to read a strong connection between war, intransigent leadership, bad governance, chaos, economic collapse, international isolation and the resultant community deprivation, with AIDS. The nagging problem, however, is that this school of thought would be immediately confronted by contradictory findings across Zimbabwe's border.

Zimbabwe's immediate south-western neighbour, Botswana, contrasts with it. Other than being a sister African country and sharing a border, Botswana is otherwise almost everything that Zimbabwe is not. Botswana never suffered any liberation wars or internal strife as was the case with Zimbabwe. Its transition from colonial rule to independence was smooth and uneventful. The country boasts one of the continent's most stable governments, an almost clockwork democratic political system, and good governance. Above all, unlike the many poverty-stricken countries of Africa, Botswana is a rich country endowed with huge precious mineral deposits among other natural resources, including vast farm land producing massive prime beef for export, and a pulsating economy that is by and large well managed. Yet by the year 2000, it was so severely devastated by AIDS that it even surpassed Zimbabwe to become one of the most affected countries in the world. In consideration of these contrasting scenarios, all that may be deduced with a certain degree of confidence is that there is much more to AIDS than meets the eye. But it would be too naïve to dismiss these sharply conflicting circumstances as unrelated to the rampant spread of AIDS for the simple reason that it happened. The prudent approach would be to examine the clues further for the missing link.

To investigate the puzzling issue of the spread of AIDS, a second visit to Uganda's border close to where it matured first presents yet another curious perspective. Uganda's giant western neighbour the Democratic Republic of Congo (DRC) presents interesting findings that may give an idea about the elusive connection. AIDS was identified in DRC at almost the same time as in Uganda. To date, some people still believe that AIDS could have spread from DRC to Rakai in Uganda; but there is no proof of that either way. The majority of the truck drivers widely assumed to have played a role in the Ugandan AIDS spread actually had DRC eastern towns as their final destination. Wars and chaos have dogged DRC from her independence from the Belgians up to the 2000s when all the neighbouring countries joined in a devastating war inside the country. The first post-independence leader, Patrice Lumumba, was brutally murdered, and a strong man, Mobutu Ssese Seko who renamed the country Zaire, ruled until he was finally thrown out. His iron-fisted autocratic reign was in many aspects comparable to that of Amin and Mugabe. Yet despite the wars, and the chaos the country has never registered HIV rates as high as most of the southern African countries which have enjoyed more tranquillity.

A detailed study of the comparative situation in various countries in order to show different levels of HIV evolvement, or to demonstrate the factors that propelled AIDS and continue to fuel it, not to mention its complex dynamics which made it so selectively devastating, are beyond the objectives and scope of this book. However, it is not always necessary to look far in order to find some useful hints. More than other continents, one may find in a single African country diverse tribal, ethnic cultures and other communities living totally different ways of life under staggeringly contrasting socioeconomic conditions. Some are even unable to understand each other's language or cultures, and are sometimes hostile or at war with each other. Uganda, for instance, has over forty recognised communities, some having much closer ancestral, ethnic or language ties with those of neighbouring countries than their fellow Ugandans. This situation pertains across the continent because the colonialists drew arbitraly borders. It is, however, not only in a cultural sense that the diversity is so apparent. It is to be found in levels of development, infrastructure, poverty and access to basic services. As varied as these are, so is the way that AIDS affected many countries.

In Uganda, it started mainly in the south-western part of the country and spread to the major towns first and then high population areas or displaced populations. Rural areas other than Rakai were initially spared and still register the lowest incidence of HIV to date, but not uniformly. Initially it looked like some tribes were immune to the disease or mysteriously spared while others appeared more prone to it. However, this was only deceptively so. A friend from the north-eastern part of Uganda once boasted in 1980s that he believed he was immune from AIDS because he thought it affected only southerners. A rude awakening came to him far too late, when he tested HIV positive. Whenever some community members moved from a low prevalence area to a high prevalence one they were affected just like the rest of the people, unless they did not integrate or lived a peculiar lifestyle. For instance, in stigmatical Lesotho, when one unfortunate foreigner was among the first to be diagnosed with HIV, while HIV was still rare there, he was unceremoniously deported, ostensibly to protect Basotho (Lesotho citizens) from the scourge. However, Lesotho went on to become one of the most AIDS devastated countries in Africa. Apparently ethnicity is not at fault but the presence of essential ingredients that constitute the AIDS bomb. It requires that essential ingredients be in place before the explosion, unless, of course, it is diffused by robust targeted interventions or exploded under controlled conditions. The HIV rates are sensitive and responsive to changing circumstances and interventions. It is those very circumstances that needed to be identified, and applied not only for better AIDS control but other emerging diseases as well.

So what do all countries that have been affected by AIDS have in common? What really fuels it? The common factor is quite obvious. Travel! It is people's movement that is the prerequisite or essential element that sows HIV in any community. The movement of tainted material like contaminated blood or blood products might have introduced the infection in some communities. However, this seems to have played an insignificant role especially in the later part of the pandemic. On the other hand, its role in the initial part wherever the original seed came from remains unclear. Travel has been a human activity since time immemorial, and virtually everyone knows that it has always been associated with epidemics of infectious diseases. Quarantines to limit human or animal movements are a prehistoric method of infectious disease control. Therefore, travel per se is too simplistic an answer to this complex question. It is perhaps more pertinent to look at travel-associated factors more closely for a better understanding of the situation. The manner and circumstances surrounding travel or migration seem to be important in the spread of AIDS, especially its effect on the cultural way of life or behaviour of the community that compounds the situation.

Among the reasons why many people in Africa have to travel include flight from wars, insurgency, persecution, famine or frequently as an attempt to escape from poverty. Their journeys are often unplanned, and chaotic, if not outright dangerous. Among them are some who have lost their loved ones or are themselves injured, with scanty possessions struggling with their exhausted, sick, starving children, fleeing from wars, as they head to the numerous bleak and cramped refugee camps. Some of the camps have turned into permanent settlements with miserable facilities in many parts of Sub-Saharan Africa. Regulated sexual behaviour is among the first things to disappear in these settlements. When I once visited a displaced people's camp in northern Uganda in 2006, I was struck by the fact that virtually all child-bearing females, including girls as young as fifteen, and a few possibly younger, had babies.

Certainly many poverty-stricken Zimbabweans desperate for work do not cross into Botswana or South Africa through the official border crossings. They must overcome numerous obstacles along their escape route including barriers, natural and manmade like electric fences, and often bribe corrupt border guards with their very last coins, before they finally arrive as penniless law breakers with no alternative but to live in the most squalid conditions as they look for jobs - any job. Often they are rounded up by the police, and deported back to their poverty stricken country. In such dire circumstances they are powerless to fight exploitation and dangerous conditions that might expose them to dangers including HIV.

However, the above portrayal does not quite fit well with circumstances pertaining to Africa's most affected country - South Africa. Since the days of apartheid, South Africa's vast mining industry has thrived on immigrant labour. Recruitment teams used to fan out into Lesotho, Botswana, and the Bantustans which the racist regime created partly as labour reserves. The massive immigrant labour force's manner of travel was well controlled and orderly. At their destination, the labour concentration camp hostels were always ready for them. Yet these people were later hard hit by AIDS. The problem here seems to have emanated from the fact that the miners were forced to live in dormitories separated from their families for long periods. This could have served as a sort of quarantine under apartheid, but when it was over there were increased opportunities for the miners to contract HIV as commercial sex workers and other women, previously banned from the areas, moved in. Not only did mini AIDS epidemics start around the mines, but the men started others in their villages when they returned to their spouses during holiday breaks. The speed at which the epidemic spread across southern African region and homogeneity cannot be explained by this phenomenon alone. This never happened in any other region of Africa. The answer at least partly swings back to travel.

To explore the effect of mode of travel on AIDS a bit further, we need to go back to a country where travel is most difficult, and then compare it to others where it is much easier. In the eastern region of the Democratic Republic of Congo (DRC) many people had to flee in disarray from marauding armed rebels. However, because the vast country lacks roads and has formidable geographical barriers and insurmountable obstacles in the form of impenetrable forests, big rivers and hostile war-lords demanding dues in different tribal areas, most population displacements and movements were by and large regionally confined. Even in peaceful areas of DRC travel remains problematic. The few overloaded passenger ferries and boats that travel on DRC's great rivers loaded with animals - including monkeys, goats and chickens - as well as foodstuffs and merchandise are as dangerous to travel on as they are a spectacle to behold. They are often the only means of travel but are used by a tiny minority of relatively well-off traders and sometimes armed gangs. For the rest of the population, countrywide movement in vast DRC is arduous, and this partly explains why the overall national HIV spread has not been as devastating as that in southern African countries where travel is mush easier.

In some isolated regions of DRC, like the eastern towns of Goma, and Kisangani, trade and movement of people are mainly to and from neighbouring Uganda and Rwanda, much more than with the rest of DRC because of the ease of access road. Likewise the HIV prevalence and disease impact is more like that of the neighbouring countries rather than other regions of DRC where the rates vary greatly. The same constraints restricted large-scale migrant labour in DRC, which, like South Africa, is a mineral rich country. However, the miners in DRC face different conditions from those in South Africa. In many mining areas of DRC there is so much insecurity that mining does not attract many people from outside the areas where they are situated. Some of the mines are run by local warlords or some powerful individuals who are a power onto themselves.

In contrast to DRC's multi-tribal country with its undeveloped travel infrastructure, Botswana, with a relatively big geographical area, has good roads and a mainly monolithic ethnic group living peacefully. HIV spread and prevalence is much higher than that of DRC despite the fact that DRC was affected first. Curiously enough all the southern African countries, whether they are rich (like Botswana) poverty stricken (like Lesotho), big in size, democratic and with economic might (like South Africa) economically devastated (like Zimbabwe), or autocratic (like Swaziland), were almost equally devastated by AIDS epidemics which seemed to spread in unison. The common factor in all these countries is a network of good roads that ensure a reliably good travel system to a common economic watering hole. All roads in southern Africa lead to Johannesburg. The people who move mostly do so for economic purposes. They are predominantly the poor, who go looking for jobs and other means of survival. This therefore tends to link poverty, ease and manner of travel or migration to the spread of AIDS in Africa.

In the year 2000 I witnessed the effect of travel on the spread of AIDS in Haiti which is inhabited by people of African ancestry. Perhaps nowhere is the association of people's movements, poverty and AIDS so easily demonstrated than in Haiti. I visited the small village town of Cange, leading a delegation of African doctors from Sub-Saharan Africa on an AIDS study tour. To get there we travelled in a high-rise four wheel drive vehicle and ahead of us was another one of the same make. Among our delegation was a Zambian lady who was so frightened by the dire road conditions and the hilly terrain that she screamed in terror every time the vehicle negotiated the numerous corners on the ragged cliffs with sharp edges. Then as we descended into a deep valley and approached a river we could to our consternation see no bridge! To our trepidation and more so the nervous lady's - who just closed her eyes - we saw the lead vehicle plunge and almost disappear into the river. Then, miraculously, we saw it emerge from the mud on the other side of the river. When we finally made it to Cange, whose only permanent infrastructure was the Catholic Church and the attached hospital, we first assembled in the church to meet with the community and some AIDS patients who had organised a community reception for us. A wonderful American man, by the name of Dr Paul Farmer, had established an AIDS care and treatment centre that was the only one providing antiretroviral therapy in the country outside Port au Prince, the capital.

We later visited some patients in their poverty-stricken village surrounding the hospital. The patients were all desperately poor, with small plots of subsistence gardens. They lived in grass thatched huts, with the exception of one patient whose tin roofed house was provided by Paul. We also met the village treatment community liaison persons called "*accompaniers*" who ensured that the patients took their medication. Virtually all patients had a few other things in common:

they had all previously "escaped" from the crushing poverty in their villages when they were well and strong and had emigrated to the tough capital city of Port au Prince to find work. Conditions in the slum areas of the city, where almost all the poor new arrivals would end up, are some of the most frightening in the world. One area dubbed Kosovo is like a battle field under the control of the mafia and is close to GHESKIO, Haiti's leading AIDS research and treatment centre, headed by Dr William Pape. Gangs of criminals specialising in drugs, sex and extortion, led by hardened godfathers, rule the slum area. I was told that even the country's police and paramilitary are scared to enter Kosovo, especially at night. Almost every morning the gangs' nocturnal work is evident in the form of bodies found dumped in various parts of the shanty town. In such dire conditions, not surprisingly, many poor job seekers from impoverished villages end up as sex workers or in situations where they are exploited sexually and become infected with HIV. As it is the survival of the strongest in the likes of Kosovo, those weakened by disease have to return home to die. Death was the fate of the vast majority of AIDS patients in Haiti, but these lucky few that I saw in Cange were saved by Paul's initiative. Virtually all early AIDS cases in Cange were those that had travelled outside the community to the capital city or abroad, while those who stayed behind were generally free of infection, until much later when inevitably the local spread started.

Travelling under duress because of poverty and dire living conditions leading to risky behaviour is an important ingredient of the AIDS bomb. However, the mere existence of these ingredients does not mean that the bomb must explode. It can be nipped in the bud. Indeed, at least one country did exactly that. Senegal started off with an epidemic that looked like it was destined to get out of hand. Yet the bomb never exploded. There was a high prevalence among commercial sex workers and the general population rate was climbing steadily towards 3% at the time when the rates in the southern African countries were also very low. Strong preventive measures focused on special risk groups, especially sex workers, nipped the epidemic in the bud. Currently the rate is one of the lowest on the continent at about 0.7%.

Uganda, on the other hand, had a very high rate of up to 30% in some sentinel sites and averaging about 15% in the later years of the 1980s and early 1990s, but strong preventive measures based on public information, education and communication leading to behavioural change as well as focused leadership brought down the rates to about 6.5%. However, it could not be brought to the Senegalese level mainly because too many people were already infected by the time effective interventions were put in place. Clearly, awareness and human behaviour seem to be responsible as secondary factors for HIV spread as well as its alleviation. Countries which did not mobilise and equip their citizens with critical unambiguous information to cause behavioural change for self-protection against AIDS fared worse. Unless risky behaviour was reduced in some other ways, like strong social or cultural etiquette that limited multiple sexual exposures.

But the dynamics of the disease point to other factors as well. The disease that started affecting mainly the well-to-do in Uganda gradually shifted to become a disease of mainly the poor or special risk groups. In USA the homosexuals were a special risk group who were able to control the new cases of the disease mainly by safe sexual practices. That is until recently, when complacency (widely blamed on too much trust in ARVs) set in reversing to some extent the gains they had made. In Uganda the rates fell fastest in towns where communication was more efficient. It seems that communication is vital in the control of the epidemic, and the lack of it to its spread.

Before leaving the relation between travel and AIDS spread, a quick review of the possible role rich Western travellers could have played in the introduction and spread of AIDS is pertinent. The Western traveller is the one that the immigration forms were designed for. Millions every year travel for pleasure and during the summer periods the airline fares are hiked and the planes fully booked by fun- seeking Western tourists. Besides sightseeing and basking under the sun on the beaches, any travel agent will confirm that sex comes in as the main, if not the ultimate, pleasure and motivator for the vast majority of young holiday travellers. In Thailand, where AIDS first matured in Asia, a lucrative industry of commercial sex workers is one of the major foreign exchange earners in an economy highly dependant on tourism. It is therefore no coincidence that it is one of the major tourist destinations of the world. In fact, at the beginning of the epidemic many of the countries dependent on tourism registered early AIDS cases. If HIV-1 was seeded in Africa from the West (as seems likely but so far remains unproven) then tourists would be the most likely carriers. Travel from the United States almost certainly introduced HIV to Haiti.

In summation, while travel and various adverse factors that promoted risky behaviour were the key ingredients of an AIDS bomb, the core dynamite of the devastating bang in Africa was and remains grinding poverty.

2
Times of Despair

Non-stop Funerals

By the early 1990s, the carnage of AIDS had made funerals in Uganda the order of the day. Tears like rivers flowed down the cheeks of shattered little children unable to bear the sight of the coffins bearing their parents' bodies being lowered into the graves, balanced on pairs of sisal strings held in position by funeral-hardened but physically-drained villagers. Parents - those that still survived, at least for a little while - fought off tears often unsuccessfully as their children, at times the very last ones, were laid to rest. Lumps filled the throats of bewildered frail old grandparents as they looked around their shanty homesteads focusing on nothing but desolation. The graveyard had rapidly expanded with graves - almost all of them dug over the previous ten years, ten years of hell. Some old dears would have made numerous journeys to the graveyard, to see off a son, a daughter, a grandchild, and the last visit for many of them merely weeks or a few months before. People grieved in different ways, according to different tribal cultures, and performed different rituals, but felt the same pain and suffered the same devastation. Their villages plunged in darkness as they watched the cream of their community perish. Yet they could see no end in sight. Funerals had become too many, too frequent, too depressing and yet they could do nothing other than watch and wait.

Ugandan, and indeed African, social and cultural etiquette, which required that everyone attends and contributes towards funeral expenses, was stretched to almost breaking point. Even if inescapable circumstances prevented one from attending a relative's, neighbour's or friend's funeral, culture dictated that one was still obliged to pay homage to the bereaved family at the earliest opportunity and also pay one's dues, known as *mabugo*.

The top carrier of the news of deaths in Uganda was the radio. A radio set could be found in virtually every parish. It was the only modern communication medium that the villagers relied on for news good and bad. In the 1960s, the newly introduced radios used to bring the villagers good news almost always in the form of music programmes and greetings from relatives living and working in towns, especially Kampala. Radios were status symbols - objects of great pleasure. Little village children, and even some mystified adults, used to steal peeps at the back of the speaking box to see the "little men" speaking from the inside. However, from the mid-1980s onwards the radio announcements programmes increasingly brought bad news. By the late 1980s the situation had turned gloomier. The radios reliably brought to the villages and from the villages to the towns more and more bad news of the deaths of friends, acquaintances or relatives, on an almost daily basis. Elderly villagers would sit around radios and many of those without sets of their own would pay a visit to the nearest neighbour, to listen to the death announcements every evening. They would sigh with temporary relief if their relatives were not among the casualties of the day but leave wondering if their luck would hold through the next day.

The death announcements became the top hit among radio scheduled programmes far ahead of all others with the only possible exception of the daily news. Often radio programmes had to be repeatedly interrupted with "breaking news death announcements" that would keep pouring in throughout the day. With the liberalisation of the media laws privately owned FM radio stations sprang up in all parts of Uganda. The private FM radio business was guaranteed instant success because of the lucrative business of deaths and funeral announcements, which often out-competed all other kinds of commercial announcements.

Following my return to Uganda from exile in late 1989, just like my fellow compatriots, I attempted to fulfil my cultural obligations. Within the first week, I was on the 390 kilometres journey on rough, potholed roads to attend a funeral ceremony of a relative who had died of AIDS. To my consternation, I was soon to realise that funerals were a very costly affair, as I had to pay for the transport, and accommodation as well as make contributions towards numerous funerals expenses. It was not uncommon to find in a village two or three burials of close relatives taking place at the same time. Occasionally two people from the same family would die on the same day, as happened to one of my cousins and her husband. Often one would be preparing to leave the village, to return to work after attending one funeral, only to be told that yet another relative had died. A friend who lived in the city once confessed that he once fled from his rural village in the middle of the night so that he could avoid further delay in the village after three consecutive days of non-stop funeral attendance. A year later and after many funeral attendances, it became abundantly clear to me that if I really wanted to do any meaningful work, and survive the journeys to and from the villages, I would need to do what the bible recommended in such circumstances: "To leave the dead to bury their own dead". But this was not always possible, especially when it came to the cases of very close relatives and friends. Even these were not few.

Despite the mass deaths, the families and various ethnic groups persevered in performing the unwieldy and expensive traditional burial ceremonies. In Uganda there are marked differences in the conduct of funerals depending on tribes, religion and regions of the country. Funerals in my home area in south-western Uganda constitute big rituals, each headed by the closest or the elder relative of the deceased. They rival weddings in pulling the crowds and bringing together friends and relatives. Among the first items to put in place is the funeral contributions record book, a basket positioned strategically at the entrance and assigned to the trustworthiest family member. The contributions range from foodstuffs, drinks, firewood, and animals to money, according to the ability and social standing of the individual. Those that may have nothing material to offer are still expected to contribute free labour to help with the funeral in any way possible. Each contribution is meticulously recorded in the book, not so much to send a thank-you note later, but rather as a sign of solidarity with the family in their hour of need. The good turn is certainly expected to deserve another at some future date when misfortune, would strike in reverse.

Traditionally, funeral ceremonies in addition to the interment of the dear departed serve many purposes. They are also occasions for grand feasts, and a bull, the size of which depends on the status of the deceased, is slaughtered. Food is prepared in abundance and drinks including commercial (if the family could afford it) and local brews served liberally. Indeed it is a great event in the villages and everyone is welcome. The burial day is a long one. The funeral has two sections, the church and the cultural parts. The church uses the occasion for long sermons, warning of the hovering death and calling upon the people to confess their sins in preparation to meet their Maker. Rarely is the topic of AIDS brought up even if it was the obvious cause of death. Instead any reference to it is indirect, and only secondary causes of death are announced. The commonest causes of death including meningitis, tuberculosis, pneumonia and others, though not always clear to the audiences, are almost always AIDS-related.

Then there are the enlogies given by the family relatives, friends, employers or workmates if the deceased was employed, local government officials and politicians. All except the politicians would shower the departed with flowery praise for the great work done while alive, even if he was just a lazy fellow. Speakers would narrate some sentimental moments shared even if the deceased was a known recluse. Everyone mentions how life would be so difficult without the dear departed one. Generous pledges to assist the bereaved family would be made, though in fact such assistance rarely materialised. The situation in general was unpleasant.

The politicians typically viewed funerals as a great campaigning opportunity. Indeed AIDS gave them many great opportunities. Huge crowds, who would otherwise never turn up to listen to politicians, would be found captured free of charge at funerals. And what should have been purely sad occasions were duly exploited for political ends. Accordingly, the politician would usually spend the shortest part of his speech on the attributes of the deceased, and swing to vote-winning strategies. The closer the elections the bigger the pledges and promises to the family the politician would make. Pledges ranged from undertaking to pay school fees for the orphans, to building the family a new house. The shattered orphans through their tears and misery would see a hazy ray of hope in their hour of wretchedness. The politician, would not miss a photo opportunity, holding the youngest of the orphans and embracing the rest of the shattered siblings.

Imagine the disappointment of the innocent, trusting chaildren when they were later sent away from school because of lack of school fees, as was frequently the case, only to realise that the promises were just a hoax. If the orphans later dared venture to approach the politician in their big offices in the city, as happened to one I know, to remind them of their pledges, many would often be subjected to a short sharp, rude rebuke, and, if they lingered around long, a kick in the backside by the security guard would be the *coup de grace*, to send them back to their non-stop misery. To be fair to the politicians, they too were faced with a very serious dilemma. The demands of the needy made much worse by AIDS among their constituents were just too many. Yet the politicians and their families were among the hardest hit by the scourge.

Other mourners had wide-ranging motives of their own. The relatives of the deceased had an obligation to attend and mental roll call of relatives is to be expected. If a close relative was absent without a very good reason then more than eyebrows would be raised. It could start a feud. The attendance of some relatives was a demonstration of innocence or denial. With widespread belief in witchcraft, some do not want to be accused of having bewitched the deceased, gloating or rejoicing at "getting rid of the deceased" in order to grab his assets, or benefit in some other way even if those are the real intentions.

Some relatives view funerals as a big family reunion, to see and meet relatives from distant places, and, in some cases, it is the only means of getting together. AIDS provided many such opportunities. The other underlying motives and reasons for attending funerals are so wide-ranging and numerous that it is virtually impossible to mention all of them. These include meeting old friends, lovers or suitors; to spite enemies; catch up on the latest rumours in the village; to get drunk or just have fun. Funerals are also an opportunity for contracting AIDS, as engaging in sexual activity is not infrequently part of it. Engaging in sex in a drunken state is a double jeopardy.

The unsophisticated villagers not related to the deceased, especially the children, usually have more down-to-earth motives for attending funerals. To many it is just a feast day and some get a chance to enjoy a rare square meal, especially the meat, and have a free drink to go with it, which they would otherwise not be able to afford. However, funerals in pre-AIDS era were never so many. There was always sufficient time in between for families to pick up the pieces and begin all over again. AIDS changed all that. Inevitably therefore the quality of the meals and the amount of foods served kept declining.

Most Africans living in cities or towns in Uganda retain a stake in a piece of land in the ancestral villages they call home. Customarily when they die their bodies are brought home for burial in the family land. The mesmerised villagers would watch awestruck as bodies of dignitaries and / or their long lost sons and daughters are brought home in shining coffins. They would stare at city people with their cars or hired vans meandering in the poverty stricken village's narrow, hardly passable, roads coming to bid farewell to one of their own, who frequently was their hope and sometimes the only lifeline, and lucky enough to have made it to the city. The close relatives in the villages would mourn the loss of gifts the departed ones used to remit to the poor home folks. Some paid school fees for their siblings and relatives, including many AIDS orphans, back in the village, who would otherwise not have gone to school. Others would be dressed in tatters if it were not for their relative in the city now being brought back to the village for burial. The source of all goodness was now gone forever.

If the deceased were married, the couples would probably have met in the city and the spouse was an alien to the village. To the relatives of the deceased, the surviving spouse would be most unpopular for two reasons. First of all, he or more likely she would be eligible to inherit the wealth of the deceased which relatives would love to grab; and, secondly, in the case of AIDS, blame would be squarely put on the survivor for bringing the killer disease to their dear departed. Never mind the fact that the reverse is more likely, since those infected longest tend to die earlier.

On a sombre note, as is usual, funerals would also be a time for grief, soul searching, and reflections, but AIDS accentuated the agony by complicating the situation further, with many more than the usual repercussions. It was especially heart-wrenching when children were involved, as was frequently the case. It is hard to bear to see grief-stricken, desperate young children at the burial of their only surviving parent, thus becoming double orphans. It is even more distressing to watch an elder sibling, a child and still in need of parental guidance, now taking over full responsibility for other younger siblings. It is depressing to watch a debilitated grandmother or a frail old grandfather trying to put on a brave face and trying to keep the devastated grandchildren together. Yet the terrible AIDS scourge brought all these to be.

Poor health, prolonged and frequent time off work to attend the funerals, over and above the increased need for food and drink to stage funeral ceremonies, as well as a reduced productive part of the population, ensured progressive poverty in society or, at the very least, the arrest of progress and development at all levels. One did not need to be an economist to see the devastation and to imagine the huge loss in productivity and development due to AIDS.

Uganda lost some of the most educated and productive people, including university professors, teachers, leading entrepreneurs, experienced managers, doctors, nurses, artists, artisans and others vital for national development. A big part of a generation of highly talented people was wiped out. As the vast majority of the deaths were between the ages of 25 and 50, which is the most reproductive age group, inevitably there were many orphans left behind, some of them infected with AIDS. The quality of education and the service sector were hard hit. Economically there were many unfulfilled projects and shattered dreams, including unfinished buildings, unpaid debts, and unrealised professional or business potential. The country, which relies on agriculture, cannot adequately describe the loss it suffered in lost productivity.

AIDS epidemic in Africa coincided with the liberalisation of politics and the economy, ushering in a new era of greater political freedom; and the collapse of apartheid in South Africa ridding the continent of the last vestiges of colonialism and institutionalised racism. It is not clear what could have been achieved without AIDS. Uganda in particular and Africa as a whole lost a golden opportunity of emancipation because of a mere bug. As for the replacement by a new generation, the prospects did not look promising The huge numbers of orphans growing up without parental guidance, and deficiency in the numbers and quality of teachers who are the natural parents' substitutes did not augur well for a robust future generation. It was back to the bleakness so well captured by the South African author Alan Paton's *Cry the Beloved Country*. Now resurrected as: *"Cry the beloved continent"*

Inevitably things started falling apart, as the cultural obligation facing unprecedented challenge clashed with modern work practices. Employers found themselves facing a serious dilemma. Absenteeism from work on account of attending funerals became unsustainable and could no longer be tolerated. Factories could no longer meet production targets; the service sector could not function smoothly; banks could no longer operate optimally; offices could not serve customers satisfactorily; patients found no healthcare providers in clinics and hospitals, and all other kinds of work that managed to go on only managed to proceed in slow motion with skeleton staff (some with skeleton figures because of AIDS) as workers attended funerals. Others were absent for a very good reason – they had died. Inevitably in that case some of the deceased's workmates would be absent for another good reason - that they were attending their colleague's funeral.

The problem for the employers was how to put a stop to all this melodrama without appearing callous and heartless in the face of the very basic human tragedy. My own organisation, the JCRC, was not spared. On November 2, 1993, My deputy wrote a letter to all staff decrying the unacceptably high numbers who were absent daily while attending funeral ceremonies of their family members and relatives. "Whereas JCRC appreciates the problem and sympathises with bereaved persons, it cannot afford to let staff go away during working hours to attend to all such ceremonies," the letter read.

To begin with, some organisations restricted attendance at funerals only to the nuclear family, but in Africa this is sensitive and not always easy to enforce without gross violation of individual privacy. A cousin is often called a brother, an uncle a father, and so on. Disincentives, including loss of wages for days off work, were tried but no method worked really well, and overall business suffered badly. Employees became poorer as they had to spend much of their income on funerals. Then demands on their remaining funds went to support orphans and dependants leaving a pittance for themselves and their own families. There was a cut in their standard of living, while demands kept on increasing as more and more relatives died. When I once told this story to a European friend he found it difficult to understand.

"Why did they not just stop? It is quite plain that it was just not sustainable and they were only succeeding in making conditions worse for their very own families" he said. Unfortunately, the situation is not as simple as that, especially as everyone considered him or herself vulnerable to AIDS and saw their benevolent action to bereaved relatives as insurance in case the same fate befell their own families. "Then in terms of development, you could as well forget it. You cannot lose so many people in their prime, and have the remainder squander their meagre resources in funerals, and still hope to beat the poverty trap," he observed, not without justification.

Well, he was right in a way, but then the alternative meant dismantling the fabric of society and its norms. The struggle to carry on regardless meant that society had to run just to keep still. But even keeping still was hard to achieve. It was more like standing still on a slow moving conveyor belt in reverse, and the full speed yet to be attained. Courtesy of AIDS.

The Opium of the Terrified

The gossip and rumour-mongering in Uganda, which started when AIDS first broke out in Rakai, had by the later part of 1980s reached epidemic proportions. Frightened people whispered about AIDS, but most of them only felt reassured enough to discuss it for as long as they were talking about others. Most conversations always ended up swinging to AIDS, funerals, the sick, the one with tell- tale signs of AIDS and so on. Virtually everyone would be talking about someone else not present. Such was the tempo of the rumours that if, for instance, a group was discussing AIDS patient X and one of them went out for a short call, the remaining group would use the absence to speculate as to whether the departing individual was sick or not.

Why were rational and usually compassionate people reduced to this weird behaviour? A plausible explanation is that they were scared by the AIDS *phobia*. This was a sort of mass hysteria triggered by the horror of AIDS and intense fear of one or more of the following: shame, blame, victimisation, guilt, ridicule, malice, injustice, disfigurement, pain, torture, and above all death. This phenomenon is often loosely referred to as stigma, though this does not adequately explain the spectrum of the feelings people had in their hearts, and why they reacted the way they did. Gossip was the opium of a distressed people trying to come to terms with the monster that AIDS had turned out to be, and to help them bear the unbearable.

Gossip and rumour-mongering were subtle forms of denial. By talking about others, people were actually saying: "It's not me, it's the other guy." This reminds one of an imaginative life insurance advertisement that said: "It is just a comforting feeling thinking that an accident will only happen to the other fellow!"

Indeed, among the people talking about the so-called AIDS "victims" were the victims themselves. It was indeed comforting for some to telecast their fears to others even if it was just for a little while, and reassure themselves that they were not bleeding inside – alone. Some patients brought up names of celebrities or prominent people known or imagined to be also infected with HIV, to make a statement that they were in good company. Chitchat lifted up the sagging morale, for a little while, and gave the sufferers courage to carry on despite the terror, hopelessness and pain of it all. But rumour-mongering also had its very negative side. It provide huge advertising media for the quacks, the con men, the profiteers peddling false hope to the sick and the desperate. Among the beneficiaries were some dubious religious organisations, as evidenced by the sprouting of highly lucrative church sects and trans-night prayers that saw their congregations, or more accurately their collections, swell. Yet the exploiters themselves were not spared.

Far from alleviating the AIDS stigma, rumour mongering on the contrary fuelled it. A big number of AIDS patients went to an extraordinary length to conceal their secret. The relatives of the patient likewise would also try their level best to keep the family "skeleton" in the cupboard. Yet, virtually all families had at least a member or a relative who had either died of AIDS or was living with it. Indeed it was taboo to say to someone's face that they had AIDS even if it was glaringly apparent.

Most doctors perpetuated the taboo by their fear and reluctance to unambiguously inform the AIDS patients and their relatives of the correct diagnosis. If a thousand medical records of the 1980s and early 1990s of patients who died of AIDS could be selected randomly, one would be lucky to find even one with a clearly written diagnosis of AIDS. Instead a new kind of jargon to mean AIDS was developed by doctors. The coined words included *immuno-suppression,* usually abbreviated as ISS, instead of *immunodeficiency,* though they mean exactly the same. The former, though, was not so readily associated with AIDS, especially if abbreviated to ISS as was most commonly the case. Evidently the doctors, just like their patients, also suffered from stigma. I remember one patient with a diagnosis of ISS excitedly explaining to friends that he had feared the worst, and yet the doctors had found his illness was in fact not AIDS. I also recall a woman getting very upset because a doctor had, in deviation of the "norm", written a diagnosis of AIDS on her brother's medical form. In another very rare departure from the practice, another doctor in a Kampala private hospital was brave enough to write the correct diagnosis of AIDS when one clergyman's oldest son died of it. The father was so incensed that he demanded a post-mortem, which was done at Mulago Hospital. It was found the son had died of *Cryptococcal Meningitis* and the old Reverend felt vindicated. In his perception and belief, he equated AIDS with immorality and did not expect his very own well brought up son to die from "fornication", as he perceived it. Yet, unknown to the cleric, *Cryptococcal Meningitis* is an AIDS-defining opportunistic infection. Sadly, worse was to follow. All his eight children subsequently died of AIDS. Years later, when death by natural causes finally put him out of his misery, he was a heart broken man. However, the tragedy was indiscriminate, and many families of all walks of life and beliefs, suffered in one way or another. Everybody knew very well that AIDS was responsible for the carnage; but when it came to individual families, it was very rarely openly accepted. It was indeed a period of mass stigma and denial.

Regarding married couples, if one came down with AIDS it was assumed and whispered that the spouse was inevitably infected. Fortunately this was not always the case. However, both the patient and the spouse would try to keep it a secret, even to their own children. I came across some puzzled HIV-infected children, asking how they could possibly have got AIDS. Some wrote heart-rending letters about their ordeal. One tearful teenage girl was crying out for an explanation, hoping that someone could believe her story that she was actually still a virgin and therefore could not possibly have AIDS. The problem here was that her mother had died while she was an infant, and the discordant father married another woman who brought her up as her own. No one had ever bothered to tell her that she had a mother who had died of AIDS and had infected her at birth. When I later asked the step-mother why she had not told the truth to the child, she evidently thought it was in the child's best interest not to know. "The child would have lived all her life in shame, knowing that her own mother was immoral," the step-mother explained. This was a case of stigma by proxy. The child was evidently one of the uncommon AIDS slow progressors to have survived to teen-age without treatment. Most children infected with HIV at birth in Africa die in infancy or early childhood.

Why some people even bothered to keep their AIDS illness a secret was just mind-boggling! It was just a vain exercise in self-delusion. It was always an open secret. Everyone who fell sick, regardless of what they came down with, was always assumed to have AIDS. Patients would make futile attempts to explain AIDS away. They would, for instance, plead that they had only fever, malaria, cough or whatever, but people would hear only AIDS. The public got to associate certain external signs and symptoms with AIDS, especially skin rashes, hair thinning or loss, inflamed lips and the dreaded shingles known locally as *kisipi*. Shingles, also known as herpes zoster, causes an acute inflammation of a nerve root and its distribution area on the skin, which gets covered with blisters that often leave scars. It also causes severe intermittent pain, which lasts long after the inflammation has healed. Whenever a patient suffered any of these signs and symptoms, even if other diseases caused it, it was always taken as confirmation of AIDS diagnosis. Many of those unfortunate enough to get shingles on the face had no alternative but to go into temporary hiding. Unfortunately, and especially when badly treated, shingles would sometimes leave unsightly scars which would be a permanent flag of sufferance and a constant reminder of the diagnosis to the public.

AIDS in Uganda was also known as *Slim* disease, because many sufferers almost always wasted away, and therefore being slim became bad news. Obesity then became a new form of denial. Some men resorted to gorging roasted fatty pork enriched by avocadoes, washed down with gallons of beer. Pork-roasting businesses flourished as it became a major weekend and evening activity. Yet AIDS had no respect for hefty fellows. Some of those who thought they could avoid AIDS by becoming fat or dating the fat, learned a "fat" lesson. One notorious Kampala paramedical quack exploited this misconception and made a fortune by treating AIDS patients with steroids. Indeed for a time, his patients appeared to improve. This was because steroids had the effect of rounding up the patients' cheeks, increasing the fats behind the neck, ballooning the tummies and generally increasing weight, but without making them better. On the contrary the steroids greatly weakened their immune system further and accelerated their demise. Later it became increasingly clear that one could have AIDS without being physically slim. While this realisation put more people on the alert, it also promoted the business of unscrupulous healers who started targeting normal looking people as potential customers for their mainly useless products.

The Face of Despair

The mid-1980s and the 1990s were bleak years for Ugandans. Horrific AIDS deaths were established as the order of the day, though no one could completely get used to the pain of it all. Each death was like a stab in the heart to anguished parents, siblings, friends, relatives and the community. Nobody knew when the nightmare would end and who would be left alive. They feared total desolation. It was very much like the bleak period of the plague of 1347 to 1350, when fear was everywhere in the air in Europe. Talking about *the Black Death* catastrophe, Giovanni Boccaccio had this to say:

> How many valiant men, how many fair ladies, breakfast with their kinfolk and the same night supped with their ancestors in the next world! The condition of the people was pitiable to behold. They sickened by the thousands daily, and died unattended and without help. Many died in the open street, others dying in their houses, made it known by the stench of their rotting bodies. Consecrated churchyards did not suffice for the burial of the vast multitude of bodies, which were heaped by the hundreds in vast trenches, like goods in a ship's hold and covered with a little earth.

Likewise in the modern era, the fear of AIDS was intense and the future outlook bleak. The priests in churches were kept busy conducting funeral services one after the other. Deaths were so many that the more popular churches had in some cases to be booked in advance. Yes - in advance! It was only that there was a new definition of "advance." If you saw the patient gasping then you rushed to send someone to book the church for the funeral service. The main churches, especially the Protestants, considering their anguished and increasingly impoverished flock, took an empathetic decision to donate the funeral services' collections to the bereaved families to help pay for the funeral expenses. Often the same pastors would have met the family a week or so before in an earlier funeral service for another family member. The battered families badly needed the money. It would indeed come in handy, especially if they were burying the family breadwinner who had spent all his worldly possessions on futile therapies to save his life. In some cases it would be the bewildered orphans burying their remaining parent. In such dire circumstances holding services in a more popular church, could mean more badly needed contributions to the bereaved family. Occasionally coffins would be lined up outside the church awaiting their turn for the service. Pastors were on duty to attend to dead AIDS victims like accident and emergency surgeons.

Nursing a patient through what became widely known euphemistically as "A long illness" would have left many families without a coin. Yet *mabugo* - funeral contributions - were no longer as generous as they used to be. People who used to be relied on to make the crucial contributions would themselves either be nursing their own relatives or would have been through a recent loss of their own. Deaths in quick successions had inevitably led to funeral fatigue. Often two or occasionally more closely related people would die at or about the same time leaving relatives in a dilemma as to which funeral to attend. Inevitably funeral attendance declined, as poverty increased. People needed money and time for other pressing priorities of life which unrelenting deaths would have made even more acute. Many people just could not be there for others because they were themselves suffering from AIDS and too weak to attend funerals. Instead they remained in bed, being helped out occasionally to sit or lie outside in the sun for a little while, to warm their shrivelled bodies, especially when there were no prying eyes around. Someone had to stay at home all the time with such a patient - to help out, and be around if he or she died. It was unforgivable for a patient to die alone without an adult family member or at least a relative in attendance to straighten the body. However, this grim task was increasingly taken over by children as adult family members decreased.

The number of strong young men who used to dig graves was dwindling, as the Grim Reaper hit their numbers hard. Villagers worried that soon bodies would pile up, as it looked like there would be no one left to bury their dead. Emergency meetings were organised in many villages, to try and find an urgent solution before bodies started piling up unburied. More grandfathers than fathers increasingly attended such meetings, as the latter's death rates were higher. It finally became clear to all that the only way the people, especially the destitute villagers, could manage the crisis was to pool their remaining energies and meagre resources together and form a rapid response burial task force to handle the deaths. They formed special village burial associations, which they named *Bataka Kweziika* translated as "citizens' self-help burial associations," to help address the predicament. Everyone was required to contribute a little money or something in kind so that help with funerals could be guaranteed for all. With the contributions hoes, shovels and other grave digging equipment were bought. *Bataka Kweziika* also helped with provision of basic logistics for the burial ceremonies, especially for the very poor or little children who had nobody else left in the family to help. The money was never enough, and the little that was there was dwindling, while funeral expenses increased. This meant that full funeral rituals were becoming unaffordable. These were replaced by abbreviated versions that catered only for the very basic needs. For instance, the funeral rites used to consist of two parts. The first part was the interment itself. The second one *"okwabya olumbe"* used to take place weeks or months later, where close relatives and friends would return to the grieving family, stay overnight, have a big feast to cleanse the home, and install the heir thus signalling the end of the mourning period. The *"okwabya olumbe"* became the first victim of the financial squeeze and was rearranged to happen with the funeral, unless of course the family could afford it.

Soon the *Bataka Kweziika* innovation became so successful that many grave diggers, who were in the past employed only occasionally, found instead that their services were needed all the time. Often the members had to divide themselves into several task forces when a number of people died at the same time. Core members became common faces, almost celebrities, as they would frequently be seen in all corners of the villages busy carrying out their grim task. In fact, the only times some would be missing were when they were sick or when they themselves were being buried by their colleagues. The *Bataka Kweziika* concept that started in the south western part of Uganda became a widespread "best" practice as a practical solution to the rampant deaths, as many other villages throughout the over-burdened country adopted it.

In the midst of this mayhem, breadwinners employed by government were losing their jobs en masse, in an insensitive but "absolutely essential" World Bank driven economic reform programme. It was dubbed 'Retrenchment', which in time became a dreaded word. In simple language it meant lay offs, dismissal or sacking. Retrenchment was a new word to many. However, the authors of the mass dismissal of public sector workers scheme preferred to call it: "Structural Readjustment", to somehow attenuate the reality of the otherwise painful exercise in more optimistic and humane terms. Whichever way one looked at it, it was still a bitter pill prescribed by the World Bank, backed by powerful economic powers; ostensibly to reform what was described as the "notoriously inefficient, corrupt and bureaucratic systems of African countries", as conditionality for further aid. Whatever its merit, retrenchment could not have come at a worse time. A considerable number of retrenched people were themselves AIDS patients. Lack of income was a sure way to hasten their death, notwithstanding their other dependant AIDS patients and the money they used to send to the villages to help out their poor folks. There were not sufficient private sector jobs to absorb the laid-off civil servants and for many the short-term prospects looked bleak. The immediate net effect for most retrenchees even without AIDS was ruin, and those with AIDS suffered a double jeopardy.

Meanwhile, the wider unrelenting AIDS scourge carried on its devastating march. Each case brought its special brand of grief to the families. Among the main special concerns of the dying was of course the after-care of their children and dependants. Those left behind were to suffer, endure hardships and deprivation in so many ways. For many children and dependants, misery would even precede the death of their sick parents. Bedridden parents could no longer provide for their children but would also spend the remaining resources in a frantic but ultimately futile battle to save their own lives.

The agony of an AIDS patient in a homestead would paralyse most family and daily life activities. It was distressing not only because of the physical pain but also the association with shame, anger, blame, fear and other psychological - aspects, including the desire to protect the family honour and to clear a guilty conscience. Among those desperate determined to protect their families' honour included one well-educated man in his late forties, holding a senior government job. He came to see me in my clinic in June 1997. He told me of his frightening plan for protection of his family from AIDS horror. As he narrated the chilling details, I was not aware that he had with him a concealed fully loaded pistol! It had all started two days earlier when he had unexpectedly reported to my clinic with puffy red eyes. He looked very tired possibly due to lack of sleep, too much drink or both. His worried expression worried me. Though I was naturally astonished to see him in that state, I was even more surprised that he specifically chose to come to me for help. The last time I had a conversation with him was way back in 1969 when we were schoolmates at King's College Budo, and we did not get on very well. The problem was that the girl he fancied at one of our school dances snubbed his advances and preferred to take to the floor with me instead. So I figured that it must be a very grave matter that would compel him to seek help from me, because over the years my repeated cautious moves aimed at a reconciliation always passed unreciprocated. Anyway, it transpired that he needed an HIV test. I went through the usual routine of pre-test counselling, taking extraordinary care to be very reassuring to him, in consideration of the ancient jealousy he once felt. I took the necessary blood samples for testing, and asked him to return for results in two days time.

That nerve-jangling Friday evening in my clinic, and looking even much more desperate than the last time, he was back to receive his HIV results. I was soon to learn that that he was just only a few hours away from putting his weapon to use. His HIV test was negative.

I had to repeat it many times before the message sank in.

"Are you playing some sort of game with me?" he demanded in a flat, disinterested voice.

"Absolutely not;" I reassured him as I brought the laboratory report closer for him to see.

He stared at it for a long time, then a teardrop materialised betraying his emotion. Wiping it away with his hand he told me of his horrific plot. It would, indeed, have been a bloody Friday. If the test had been positive, he had planned to die with his entire family. Thrusting his hand in his inner jacket pocket, he pulled out a document. It was his suicide note. He stared at it for a moment as he shook his head, and then tore it up and threw the pieces into my dustbin. Collapsing in the chair with tears freely flowing down his cheeks he grieved over his ordeal.

"My girlfriend died of AIDS," he sobbingly said. "I thought I was infected too and in turn feared that I had infected my wife, and she in turn the children," he explained between wiping the tears from his face. "Images of disfigurement, pain and torture of my wife and my children, as I watched helplessly, kept reverberating in my mind days on end until I could take it no more!" he said sobbingly. "Recently it has been like a horror movie playing over and over again," he added, his composure improving a little. "I agonised over suicide but I could not leave the family to suffer. The only way I could see was just to put me and my entire family out of the shame and misery of AIDS." Still wiping away the tears with self evident embarrassment, he added: "You see, doctor, I was just not thinking right any more. I was desperate. Oh God! How I have suffered with worry over the years," he moaned. "I wish I had the courage to do this earlier. I would not have lived this nightmare for so long"

As a mainly sexually transmitted disease, AIDS is like a chain reaction. First of all it normally takes two for it to occur. Men and women infect each other. Husbands infect their wives and the wives in turn infect their children. In those tribes which practise widow inheritance, the infected widows infect their new husbands and the reaction goes on. Therefore, the usual sequence of sad events was such that as hope fades for the individual victim, worried consideration would shift to those next in line on the chain of death. These would be the spouse, offspring, mistress or some other sexual contacts. The very thought of going through the same ordeal all over again would send shivers down the spine of everyone within the extended family, especially those personally concerned.

In Uganda and Africa at large, women are the family and community nurses. They patiently stay by the bedside of the sick, attending to their needs, enduring even if conditions worsen until the patients succumb and die in their arms. In the peasant subsistence economy of Uganda, and indeed most of Africa, the same women also play a crucial social economic role. Their absence from family gardens and other income-generating activities, while nursing the sick, had great but not always visible adverse socioeconomic implications, ranging from insufficient food production and malnutrition to failure to sustain children at school, and predisposition to diseases (including AIDS itself). Most men, on the other hand, usually not as good for emotional support, stay by the bedside for only a short time and render help from a distance.

A typical scenario around the death-bed is that of women gathered around while the men folk squat in the compound or sit in the waiting area talking in low voices, unless alcohol changes the mood. Meanwhile the baffled children trying to make sense of it all are left wondering in between. Friends, neighbours and relatives move in and out of the house all day long and a few close ones come to stay. However, in extreme cases, as a result of stigma some relatives shield the AIDS patient from all except a few trusted friends. This sometimes subject the patient to further pain and suffering with no psychological support. This bewilderment goes on until the patient die.

Nonetheless, the human spirit is often indomitable. In the midst of chaos and hardships, many devastated dependants somehow rise, find a new level, pick up the pieces and carry on. The more heartbreaking examples involved children. As we opened one rural AIDS treatment centre I met a twelve year old who had single-handedly brought up his sister from the age of two following the death of their parents. The problem was that he was in the terminal stages of AIDS and would soon die without antiretroviral drugs. His sister was also infected but was not in advanced stage of the disease. We were able to help both of them but this was by no means either the only such case or the worst example.

The businesses or assets left behind by deceased parents were often stolen from the children, or taken over by either inexperienced relatives or mismanaged by caretakers who did not have the same skills, interests or stamina as the departed ones. I recall a case of a fairly prosperous patient who instead of paying for life-saving antiretroviral treatment decided, against advice, to die and leave his estate to his children, arguing that he did not want to leave his children in destitution by spending all the money on the then very expensive therapy. After his death, his property, as is common in Africa, was uninsured and unregistered and was lost because of a small debt. Most of my patients who remained alive by investing in ART always did better for their families in the end despite the drugs costing them so much. The vast majority, however, just could not find any resources to pay for the exorbitant drugs. Nevertheless, for all those who could somehow afford the life-saving therapy, I made sure that treatment was always available at the Joint Clinical Research Centre. In addition, I adopted a strategy to ensure constant surveillance of the drugs market to identify sources of lower cost quality drugs, so that I could continually increase both access and the numbers of lives saved. Another serious constraint was the social security system and child safeguard laws, which were too weak to offer legal protection for the orphans and dependants. Legally binding wills and insurance schemes were rare and, in any case, no insurance company was willing to offer policies to AIDS patients. Governments in Africa, cognisant of the huge bills involved, kept blinkers on as far as antiretroviral drugs were concerned, though clearly it was the most cost-effective way to reduce the carnage and the orphan problem, by keeping patients alive as long as possible.

Indeed, the future for Uganda and Africa in general looked depressing. Right from the family unit, up to national level, the agony was palpable as the epidemic continued to wreak havoc. Not surprisingly, once at a big public gathering in Bushenyi, southern Uganda, where I was officiating at the opening of an AIDS treatment clinic, I asked the congregation to indicate by a show of hands if they had lost at least one family member to AIDS and secondly, if there was at least one AIDS orphan in their households. All hands shot up in response to both questions. As the hands lingered in the air, I thought I could discern expressions of bewilderment, which quickly turned to resignation as everyone looked around and realised that they were not alone - everybody was obviously bleeding inside. AIDS was a mass disaster, causing mass misery. And there was uncharacteristic silence. There were no spare shoulders to cry on. No one to turn to for commiseration. Everybody with his own sorrows, and too mortified to bother the neighbour overburdened with his own.

Uganda was losing the cream of her society to AIDS, leaving behind helplessly destitute orphans and a traumatised impoverished population. Clearly, AIDS was annihilating a generation, as the antiretroviral drugs that could have averted more deaths were denied to the dying: on account of their poverty.

Heartbreak Orphans

As the carnage due to AIDS involved mainly people in their reproductive years, the number of orphans literally exploded. By the year 2000 the situation had deteriorated, not only in Uganda where AIDS orphans were estimated to have surpassed the one million mark, but also across the Sub-Saharan region, especially in southern Africa where the epicentre of the epidemic had shifted to. UNAID estimated the numbers of children globally who had lost one or both parents to AIDS to have reached about 14 million, and projected that if nothing was done the numbers would jump to a shocking 25 million by 2010. Of these orphans a staggering 80% were Africans, who, incidentally, constitute only 10% of the world population, thus underscoring the serious magnitude of the problem on the African continent. Meanwhile, in 2002 the children infected with HIV in Africa were conservatively estimated to number about 2 million and still rising rapidly. Despite the very high death rates the numbers were projected to rise to well over 3 million by mid 2005.

Thanks to the African culture, almost all orphans were initially absorbed within the traditional system where they found shelter and with care from blood relatives. Blood relationship in Africa is often almost as close as parental relationship. Sometimes it can be so close that the children do not even know that the caretakers are in reality not their biological parents. But that was before the AIDS scourge strained the tradition. When the going got tough, and food became scarce in some homesteads, the biological children were prioritised over the orphans. Whenever the food was scarce, then hapless orphans would sleep hungry despite the fact that more often than not, the older ones among them would have prepared the meal. Some orphans were in effect more like house helps. In situations of childhood rivalries and competitions, almost inevitable in most homes, the orphans would not stand a fighting chance. Thus, in almost all important family matters, even those that directly affected them, orphans would often find themselves on the outside looking in. Even under such tough conditions those that had shelter and some sort of care were the lucky ones.

The children's uncles and aunts are culturally the first line relatives to take over care of orphans following the death of their parents. Initially, an uncle or aunt would take in all the orphans from the same family, thus giving the siblings a chance to grow up together and bond as brothers and sisters. However, as more and more relatives died it became impossible to keep all the siblings together, and therefore a practice of sharing out the children among several relatives started. Sadly, this meant that siblings would be almost strangers as they grew up.

As no one was immune from the marauding AIDS epidemic, some orphan caretakers also became victims. Indeed, the good uncles and aunts, being of the same generation as the orphans' late parents, were themselves among the highest AIDS risk group. As many of them died, their own children plus the foster orphans for the second time round would be on the move. If there were no more uncles and aunts alive or able to take the orphans in, then the mantle would be passed on to some more distant relatives. Yet the more distant the relationship was with the orphans, the less the attachment. The poor children would be looked at more like a burden of problems than a bundle of happiness. The distant relatives would be less inclined to go the extra mile and make the necessary sacrifice for them over and above their own pressing problems, sometimes including responsibility of caring for more closely related orphans. Meanwhile, one other traditional door, albeit controversial, that provided care to orphans within the same family set up was being slammed shut by AIDS. It was the traditional practice of widow inheritance, which was previously a common practice. Dr Ntozi, a Ugandan researcher, found that as early as 1995, widow inheritance had sharply declined in Uganda due to the fear of AIDS. In addition, AIDS made remarriage of victims (which was another way of giving some sort of stability and a secure home to orphans) problematic.

In the midst of this mayhem, the only adult relatives of the wretched orphans with low death rates from AIDS were the grandparents. The grandparents, often old widows as women tend to outlive their husbands, were left with no alternative but to take on the homeless and helpless orphans who had no younger relatives left or willing to take them on. Some of the orphans were infants or even occasionally just newly born as some mothers weakened by AIDS would not survive childbirth. Stories of some very poor grannies - with no other possible source of infant food - resorting to breast feeding their grandchildren were not uncommon. Sheer desperation would drive them to reactivate their shrivelled breasts to perform the motherly function one more time in their twilight years.

The elderly Ugandan, and indeed most African old timers, unlike those in developed countries who survive on pension or social security, looked forward to their own children supporting them in their old age. Yet AIDS robbed them of their life insurance – their own children. The vanquished grandparents lived miserably deep in the villages feebly scratching the earth and foraging as they waited only to meet their maker. Yet the same cruel AIDS scourge was calling upon them, or rather forcing them, to arise once more and take up the mantle of feeding, providing and educating their grandchildren at the time when their physical energies and resources were all but drained. The situation kept deteriorating for many of them, as more and more children kept coming to them.

However, even with these cultural contingency measures in place, the saturation point was soon reached, and a new situation previously unknown in African culture emerged;homes headed by children. In some of the worst reported cases, six year-olds took over responsibility for their younger siblings, foraging and scavenging for them as best they could. The situation was so desperate for some orphans that even those who had elder siblings to look after them were relatively lucky. Some children, just toddlers, found themselves without homes or anyone to look after them. Some just gravitated to the streets and became known as the "Street Children." The population of street kids in Uganda had risen as a result of previous social turmoil due to wars and bad governance, but from the mid 1980s onwards it swelled rapidly and was mainly fuelled by AIDS.

Some orphans suffered even worse ordeals. One East African newspaper reported the dreadful story of an orphan in Kenya, who, following the death of his mother, was locked in the house with her corpse by stigmatised, superstitious and terrified villagers leaving the child to die a slow death. Fortunately the grim story spread rapidly and the child was rescued by a charitable organisation, which kindly buried the rotting body of the mother, which the villagers had feared to touch.

Many of those who took on orphans endured severe strain on their meagre family resources. As a result, the children suffered increased malnutrition, which in turn made them more vulnerable to diseases. Needless to say, many orphans' caretakers found it virtually impossible to provide them with other basic needs. Among the most unfortunate orphans were those who had AIDS passed on to them by their mothers. Children born with AIDS in Africa had a nightmare of a life characterised by painful recurrent infections which tortured them. Without AIDS drugs they would have required antibiotics and painkillers to give them even temporary relief. Yet even these palliatives were not available or accessible to many. As a result the vast majority of orphans and poor children with AIDS just had to suffer the pain, until death put them out of their misery. Arguably, the silver lining (or should it be lead lining) in this sad episode was that for many, death was relatively quick as the majority of children who acquired AIDS from their mothers died in infancy or early childhood.

Gone were the good old days when it used to be said, "Africa has no orphans." Virtually all of them would be incorporated into the relative's families, but AIDS changed all that. The sheer numbers just overwhelmed the traditional practice as the smaller numbers of survivors could not cope with the demand. Then, finally, the phenomenon of orphanages that I read about in Charles Dickens' books, that were alien to Uganda, mushroomed in many parts of the country. Most of the orphanages were started by foreign charity organisations that were soon joined by some local non-governmental organisations (NGOs). Institutional care and support therefore became an alternative source of assistance to orphans. Like in the days of Oliver Twist, the boy in the Charles Dickens' book, some of the orphanages set up supposedly to help AIDS orphans were just terrible. Some were set up by unscrupulous people with ulterior motives mainly to capture donor aid funds for themselves. Therefore some of the orphans who were unlucky to find themselves in such an unfortunate situation were used more like hostages. Fortunately, the rest of the orphanages were a God-sent blessing to the small numbers of lucky orphans who found room there.

A 1997 report indicated that most orphan aid programmes in Uganda provided only basic needs and school fees, but evidently these services reached only a tiny minority. Those with AIDS just died, as the carers could do nothing about it. It was not until free AIDS therapy for some patients in Uganda became available in 2004 that carers started to have some means of treating orphans with AIDS.

Some NGOs with grants for the care of orphans occasionally made unintended blunders that only served to make the sad conditions even worse. I was told a disheartening story concerning a group of workers from one foreign NGO who visited an inner city slum area in search of destitute orphans to enlist on their programme in order to render them some assistance. Coming to one makeshift home, loaded with goods Father Christmas style, they asked whether there were orphans.

"Yes" was the answer.

As I later confirmed they could have heard the same answer from almost the all the ramshackle abodes. The respondent was reportedly a haggard middle-aged woman who supported her family selling homemade cookies by the nearby roadside. She and her unemployed husband were taking care of two orphans as well as four other children of their own.

"We have two orphans with us. They had no one else to turn to. So we took them in" she explained.

"Do they have blankets?" one of the NGO workers asked.

"No."

"Do they go to school?"

"No, we could not afford school fees."

"Great, what are their names, and ages?" The NGO worker purportedly asked as she reached for the big register book and pen. "We shall pay their school fees, and provide them with meals," she added.

Then the big bag was brought forward as all the other children in rags stared agape in amazement at the bountiful contents.

However, only two blankets, two shirts, and two pairs of shorts were given out to the incredulous two orphans while the rest of the children stared on green with envy. But the donors still had something more to say, which could have made the other kids think that being an orphan was after all not such a bad thing.

"As the orphans are now registered, we shall from now onwards be coming over to monitor their progress and to provide for their needs," they announced to the foster parents, as they prepared to leave to repeat the same exercise in the next tumbledown dwelling.

What these well meaning benefactors did not immediately realise were the dire circumstances endured by all children in the home. They all lived and shared the same miserable conditions. The added burden of orphans in their destitute family had made their dire situation much more miserable. All the children spent nights huddled together trying without success to keep warm in the dilapidated dwelling as they all had no blankets. Reportedly only two of the other children were going to school. Now the causes of their increased misery were being rewarded and they the double victims, were excluded. It does not take much imagination to visualise what the atmosphere in the shanty home must have been like after the departure of the naive donors.

I learned more about the dire circumstances faced by orphans in 2003, when I was commissioned by UN-HABITAT to study the orphans' situation in the inner city slums of Mulago and Kamwokya areas of Kampala. My three research assistants and I spent over six months visiting the swarming slums. We witnessed the filthiest conditions imaginable. I literally stared poverty and suffering in its ugly face. The so-called houses where the orphans lived had minimal or no basic toilet facilities, and provided little privacy if at all. Outside the houses, the environment, provided no or minimal refuse management resulting in rotten, smelly, fly-and pest-infested heaps of garbage. Human and animal excreta added to the environmental risk for infections. Starving dogs and occasional stray cats scavenged on the refuse but, obviously by their appearance, and like the poor children, not finding much. Not surprisingly, cholera and dysentery outbreaks were common. Just before the survey, the areas had been under quarantine to control an outbreak of cholera. There were almost no access roads and to go in one had to jump over wide ditches, mini-rivers of filthy water from numerous slum dwellings with raw sewage floating along. Needless to say, most of the makeshift homes lacked even the basic necessities of life like food and clothing. All I could see inside were a few scattered rags. The net effect of these awful conditions resulted in increasing numbers of children spilling onto the streets as beggars, pick pockets, drug peddlers, juvenile prostitutes, drug addicts and committers of other more serious crimes.

Virtually every slum dweller, perhaps with the exception of criminals who used the area as a hiding place from justice, was miserably poor. But the poorest of the poor were by far the orphans we found there. There were also disturbingly high levels of child labour and exploitation. Orphans in particular were used as household help doing daily chores, including fetching water from distant sources mainly wells, which were not always protected. Young children carried on their heads heavy 20 litre jerrycans of water, and did adult household work including cleaning, cooking, washing clothes, taking care of siblings or baby-sitting for others. Some also worked as housemaids for free or for a pittance at best, and for long hours. Orphans were most vulnerable to other kinds of abuse, including sexual and physical assaults. They were also often victims of petty and serious crimes, which were the order of the day in the slums.

Schooling and education opportunities were greatly reduced especially for orphans despite an official policy of "free Universal Primary Education" (UPE). The programme did not provide all the requirements for schooling. UPE in Uganda is in reality a partnership between government and parents whereby the parents are expected to provide meals and clothing and also make some contributions towards buildings and maintenance while the government covers school fees. These requirements are the reasons most orphans dropped out of school. Other reasons include exploitation by caregivers who selfishly keep them at home as house aids, or to take care of the sick within the home, as well as lack of guidance.

In the slums I found that non-governmental organisations, community-based organisations and faith-based organisations were conspicuous by either their absence or the minimal roles they played. The few that I could clearly identify did not appear to make much impact because they were under-funded, poorly managed, lacked focus, uncoordinated, or just bogus. It was clear to me that most services claimed by these organisations did not always trickle down to people who needed them most. For those targeting HIV/AIDS, it was common to find that they had no specific policies in place for orphan and vulnerable children (OVC), and at best just participated in HIV/AIDS awareness in a vague sort of way.

The main day-to-day torturer of orphans in the slums was by far hunger. The children were just starving. All the people we interviewed, including orphans themselves, identified food as the immediate need of orphans and vulnerable children. This of course would not be surprising to the readers of *Oliver Twist* because the situation that existed then in Europe was reborn over a century later in Africa, but in much harsher conditions. The second priority need that I identified was medical care followed by a list of others. Among the disturbing findings was the direct physical hardship which the orphans also suffered. Most slum shelters had leaking roofs and whenever it rained, especially at night, the children would be soaked. Most had no blankets or other form of beddings, and space was so scarce that some slept in turns. This, of course, applied to all children in the slums irrespective of whether they were orphans or not. However, the orphans' situation was worse and in turn made the bad condition of other children worse. Evidently AIDS was clearly one of the leading causes of the worsening poverty.

I found that many female children who drop out of schools ended up getting married at a very early age. There were many teenage pregnancies, and the consequent complications that go with it, as well as a worsening of an already bad social situation. There was also sexual corruption of children. Due to limited space, teenagers shared rooms with their single mothers who were some times cohabiting, hence their sexuality tended to be activated at an early age which greatly increased the risk of acquiring AIDS.

Orphans and vulnerable children also suffered other serious disasters as a result of dismal slum conditions, including vector-borne and communicable diseases, injuries arising out of crammed conditions and violence, not excluding rape. At a very basic level the OVCs miss out on the very few available social services including immunisation and access to primary healthcare. Generally theirs was a life of misery, and uncertainty. When caretakers died in the slums some of the orphans had nowhere to go except the villages where they faced equally harsh or worse conditions. Ironically the traffic was bi-directional, as some of those already in villages who lost their carers were often shipped to the slums to stay with the remaining relatives living there.

It became quite clear to me as I worked in the slums that unless the marauding spread of HIV was addressed the orphan numbers would keep on growing and the problem would become much more complex. The most plausible action required to quickly tackle the creation of

AIDS orphans was to provide affected parents with the life-saving AIDS drugs. The power of AIDS drugs to drastically decrease the death rates had been clearly demonstrated by Brazil's universal ART access programme. In fact, it put a sudden stop to massive deaths in Brazil when it was introduced. Furthermore, as far as AIDS sick orphans and vulnerable children were concerned, they were clearly the poorest of the poor and needed to be the priority group to access free ART, as they had no possibility of fending for themselves. I considered their plight to be of critical moral and ethical imperative. When my centre obtained free drugs through PEPFAR funding I made sure that orphans and vulnerable children were the first to access this life-saving therapy.

However, fully aware of the multiple problems that face orphans and vulnerable children with AIDS infection, I realised that they could not live by the drugs alone. There was still a lot to be done to make a meaningful difference to their pathetic lives. Despite the fact that AIDS cut across the entire society, orphans (especially those who had AIDS) were the very poorest of the poor. They needed priority consideration and special help if they were to stand a chance to grow up as responsible citizens. Yet either too little help or none at all was forthcoming.

Voodoo Cures

In September of 1989, all roads leading to a sleepy village of Nkutu in Ssembabule, in Masaka district of Uganda, were jammed with traffic, more so the main southern highway from the capital city, Kampala. The jam was in both directions. The multitude of vehicles - far above the usual traffic - were either heading to or returning from the same place. At the centre of it all, the atmosphere in the village that had never witnessed the like in its history was highly charged, almost like a fanatical pilgrimage site. Most of the vehicles involved in the commotion, mainly taxi minibuses, had a number of things in common. First of all, they were all full of hyper-excited people, some waving tree branches through the open windows, some chatting loudly and others just singing merry songs. No one seeing these people in such euphoric state could have imagined that any one of them was at death's door or that they suffered great psychological trauma. Many vehicles on their return leg were decorated with tree branches as if they were returning from a wedding or an exciting event. Almost everyone was in celebratory mood like soccer fans returning from a victorious away match against their bitterest rivals. Whenever the vehicles travelling in opposite directions met whistles would be blown, "V" signs flashed out and tree branches waved. The home-bound would urge those going to hurry, and those still on their way to the venue would feel envious of those returning.

"*Fe tufunye ebyaffe*" those on the return leg would shout, meaning, "We have already got our share!"

Those on their way would shout back: "*Naffe katonda atuyambe tufune*" "Please God help us to also get ours too" Encouraged, but worried that the whole thing could all be over before their arrival, the passengers would urge the drivers to speed up and take them to their salvation.

The unprecedented crowd-puller was the mud and wattle home of one elderly illiterate, devout Catholic peasant village woman by the name of Nanyonga. She had just pulled off what was described as a "miracle." News about the sensation in Nkutu village had spread far and wide like wild fire. It touched on a very sensitive nerve of very desperate people, offering hope where there was only gloom. They flocked in from all corners of Uganda, and some came from the neighbouring countries of Tanzania, Rwanda, Zaire (now DRC), and Kenya. The specific cause of the excitement and commotion was that word had spread that Nanyonga had found a cure for AIDS. People talked about her as if she was a saint, and whispered about the miraculous qualities of her medicine and the thousands of people she had cured. The numbers she reportedly restored to health varied widely but consistently kept increasing the farther the distance from Nkutu. Almost 200 kilometres away in Kampala, they talked of hundreds of thousands. Anyone who appeared to doubt the genuineness of this great news would be shunned or verbally chastised. Many desperate people, for the first time since the carnage started, seeing a ray of hope, mobilised all their resources and rushed to get their share of the magic potion before it all vanished, as the demand was evidently very high and rising still.

At Nanyonga's home the rush would turn into a stampede as people jostled and shoved to get their share of the miraculous medicine. However, there was an inescapable catch and some crucial regulations that made the hold-up inevitable. The bottleneck resulted from the critical need to follow the protocol essential for ensuring the effectiveness of the cure. Apparently, the miracle medicine would only work if the one and only Nanyonga dispensed it in person. Secondly, the medicine would not work unless the sick person received it personally. In addition, the wonder medicine would also immediately lose its healing powers if it were sold. Nanyonga herself never charged a penny for it.

At its peak, the queue of expectant patients was said to stretch for up to three kilometres. Although almost the entire frantic crowd consisted of AIDS patients, the drug itself according to Nanyonga was in fact a panacea - that cured all diseases! The huge crowds attracted a considerable number of vendors who saw some business opportunities and set up makeshift shops selling drinks, roasted meat and bananas. Despite the stern warning that the medicine would lose potency if sold, some incorrigible opportunists still sought to commercialise the so-called medicine and reap very high profits. It was all like a gold rush. However, in this case they needn't have worried too much. The valued product was available in such huge amounts that it was virtually inexhaustible. By the time Nanyonga closed shop, she had dished out a staggering thirty tons of it.

According to Nanyonga, the chosen one, the miraculous medication was revealed to her in a vivid vision that occurred while she slept one momentous night, September 8, 1989. That fateful night, a blinding flash of light and a powerful commanding voice, which according to her could only be that of God, heralded the discovery. "Go forth Nanyonga," the voice of God reportedly instructed her, "and cure all diseases!"

The revelation directed her to the exact spot where the bountiful medicine was, and instructed that only she could collect it and dispense

88   *Genocide by Denial*

it otherwise it would be inactivated. Fortunately, she did not have to go far to reach the wonder medicine. It was right there in her backyard. As for the medicine itself, it was – wait for it - soil! By the blessed magical touch of Nanyonga, ordinary soil would immediately be transformed into a potent panacea that cured all diseases including the dreaded AIDS.

Gossip, not denied by Nanyonga, had it that the first one to benefit was no other than her own niece, Margaret Nazziwa. One Ugandan newspaper reported that she was on the verge of death and bedridden in a Kampala hospital. As soon as she partook of Nanyonga's medicine-soil mixed with cold water she miraculously recovered. For a time she was right there frolicking for everyone to see, but this newly-found lease of life did not last long as she later died suddenly. Nanyonga explained away her niece's death as having been caused by "lack of faith." Yes. One had to have faith in the magical powers of her medicine in order to benefit from it.

The hole in the ground that started as a scratch on the surface was soon transformed into a huge crater as Nanyonga shovelled out tons and tons of the soil and dispensed it to the throngs of people. Although the soil medicine was free it was whispered that whoever wanted to leave anything would not be in breach of the rules, but Nanyonga never openly canvassed for donations.

The bemused Ugandan Ministry of Health (MOH) got wind of a woman that was outshining them and putting them out of business. Many AIDS patients had voted with their feet, abandoning the hopelessness and desperation of the MOH hospitals manned by doctors with nothing better to offer. AIDS patients escaped these death houses, which the hospitals, without any effective medicine for AIDS or credible palliative, had turned out to be. They made a beeline to the new beacon of hope that did not merely offer advice on "living positively" but promised them a cure. Meanwhile, the Ugandan press was awash with Nanyonga stories that captivated the AIDS-battered population and indirectly became Nanyonga's client mobiliser. The MOH came under severe criticism from the restless public for failure to come out boldly with a clear statement to confirm that the medicine really worked. Such was the extent of desperation in the country that many just did not want the Ministry of Health to extinguish the only beacon of hope, however far fetched it was. It was the only hope that many tormented suffers at the end of their tether could see.

The Ministry of Health should have had no difficulty in coming out with a clear statement about the chaotic situation. In fact, they did not have to make any statement at all. All they needed to do was to ring the nearest police station and ask them to urgently go over to Nanyonga's compound and read the riot act to the hoodwinked crowd. On the contrary, and most incredibly, the MOH formed an investigative committee. They trailed their own deserting patients all the way to Nkutu village, to see and assess how the miracle treatment worked out for them. What they found there just shocked them. They found thousands of people who were just consuming soil dug up by a perspiring, old woman. Nanyonga did not seem healthy herself, and the soil was being dispensed in the most unhygienic conditions imaginable. Obviously this had to be stopped immediately. However, the delegation read the mood of the mammoth crowd correctly. If anyone dared tell the hyper-excited crowd that their only lifeline was nothing but ordinary soil, he or she would be lynched. Prudently, the MOH officials made a tactful retreat to the safety of their headquarters in Entebbe, on the shores of Lake Victoria, and then blew the whistle on Nanyonga.

Incredibly there were some people, who vehemently argued that the soil should have been subjected to scientific tests to see whether it had magical healing powers against AIDS or not! In the aftermath, the question many people asked in reflection of the four weeks of brisk soil consumption was: how could so many people, including some highly educated ones, be so foolish? This question is perhaps best put to a rescued drowning man, who held on to a straw. Such was the desperation of AIDS.

However, this was not the only absurd scenario. Frantic people trying to escape death are easy to deceive. Rational thinking tends to be relegated to the background as the terrified cling on to every word of hope, however fanciful. They look for a solution in everything, and see hope in shadows. It is easy to believe that this only happens in Africa, or to this or that group of people; but when faced with such despair I have seen virtually all peoples of every culture, race and background behaving in the same way or worse.

As we launched a new antiretroviral therapy centre in the south western town of Ibanda, early 2006, the guest of honour was Monsignor Muntu. In his speech, the Catholic cleric referred to a time of despair way back in mid 1980s when dogs almost became extinct in the area. The dogs' misery stemmed from yet more bizarre gossip that circulated in the neighbouring villages, that dog's soup cured AIDS. No one knew, how, when and where the gossip started. In Uganda dogs are not used for food. However, the situation in neighbouring Democratic Republic of Congo (DRC) is different, because in a few areas dog's meat is a delicacy. Therefore, some speculated that the gossip started from DRC.

In 1987, the period of utter desperation, an Egyptian quack appeared who had teamed up with a Congolese who both caused quite a stir when they claimed to have discovered an AIDS cure from their "research" carried out in Egypt and the Democratic Republic of Congo. They named their so-called "wonder drug" *Mubarak-Mobutu* cure, presumably in "honour" of the presidents of their two respective countries. Their so-called medicine, which they administered by injection, was extremely dangerous. It caused a high fever in many of the recipients. It could have infected some of those uninfected with AIDS, and made those already infected worse. It was rumoured that these two men got hold of infected blood and separated plasma from it, and then just half boiled it and used it to inject patients. Worse still, it was also promoted as a possible vaccine to be used among the uninfected to prevent HIV. Fortunately they were stopped in their tracks but not before the Egyptian made all kinds of wild allegations and accusations against the Ministry of Health officials. He also claimed that it was the CIA and other imaginary enemies out to stop him from saving the lives of poor Africans.

In summary, there were many other voodoo healers from all walks of life and professions, including physicians, whose absurd stories would fill a book. They include a Ugandan quack who caused a sensation in the country when he peddled an ordinary vitamin C concoction, named after his mother, as a potent AIDS medicine, and a Kenyan professor who peddled a food supplement all over East Africa as an AIDS cure. There were also some useless so-called herbal "AIDS cures" marketed by self-styled herbalists who made a fortune, before some of them succumbed to the grim reaper themselves.

Even when AIDS patients weakened and wasted away most of them and their relatives still hoped for some miraculous remedy. They frantically looked everywhere for a cure in vain, but many of them never lost hope until the very hour of reckoning.

When the Vultures Come Flying In

I met some distraught terminally-ill patients, praying that death would mercifully come sooner rather than later to put them out of their misery. On their deathbed, AIDS patients were magnets for all kinds of visitors, including intruders with diverse motives, not always honourable or inspired by compassion. The assortment included healthcare providers, traditional healers, herbalists, witchdoctors, spiritual healers (bona fide and quacks), as well as people who just come to watch events as they unfolded. Con men and opportunists hoping to snatch a share of the spoils before it was snatched away were among them, under the pretext that they are trying to help. The family, out of desperation, often pool their dwindling resources to pay for all sorts of concoctions, rituals and prayer supposed to help. Yet in the deepest of their hearts, almost everyone knew very well that AIDS had no cure, and that the victim would die. Yet many still believed that some divine powers, or someone, somehow, could conjure up some magic that would make their loved one an exception.

Meanwhile, the entire commotion constitutes a nightmare for the doomed patient, so much so that the inevitable demise almost seem; like a welcome relief. Many patients do not even get a wink of sleep. Yet in their excruciating pain, sleep was what many yearned, because it was the only relief that worked for them for however short. Whoever turned up claiming to have a remedy would be ushered in to see the ill-fated victim, in the hope that he or she would wave the magic wand. Even what could have been a welcome moment of quiet during the night would often be brutally disrupted by raucous night prayers that sprang up as an epidemic of its own reflecting the increasing desperation in the community. Meanwhile some of the relatives would be on wild goose chases following up grapevine talk of healers and drugs.

Herbalists opened up numerous clinics and advertised themselves and their useless cures extensively. Their agents would keep their ears close to the ground identifying homes with dying patients to target! In a rush to cash in on the bonanza, some people abandoned their jobs, professions and businesses for the new and more lucrative money-spinning business of "herbalism." Not to be out competed, those in the spiritual business responded by establishing numerous makeshift churches and forming new religious sects, specially targeting the huge clientele of terrified AIDS patients and their families, offering them miraculous spiritual cures and deliverance. Some AIDS patients, without hope and resigned to the inevitable doom, were easily persuaded to join and seek solace. Like the herbalists some religious sects also had agents to visit and pray for the sick for a fee, as well as persuade the relatives to either carry the sick to the churches or attend on their behalf. Many sects specialised in all night prayers. The prayers were usually led by self-styled, pastors accompanied by deafening drumming and singing aired over powerful sound amplifiers. The noise only stopped briefly from time to time for collections while chanting the likes of, "Give generously to the Lord, to thank him for casting out the devil out of this patient, so that he can in return reward you abundantly."

Some opportunistic sects perfected the art of cheating patients and their relatives. This included the abolition of anonymous offerings, and replacing it with a system whereby all donations had to be clearly displayed for all to see. Others did away with all small change offerings.

These persuasive confidence-trick pastors would in various ways keep hinting at or emphasising that God's reward depended on the amount of money donated. "Oh, God is not worth a mere one thousand shillings. Imagine all the blessings. Suppose he reciprocated in the same way," some pastors would recite, as they worked up the crowds of worshipers. "God knows how much money everyone has in their pockets. If the blessings fall short, it is not because I did not pray hard enough for you, but it is simply because you did not reciprocate his abundant favours adequately."

One church-going widow who lost her husband to AIDS but was herself not infected told me of her ordeal. Following the sudden death of her son, one greedy self-styled pastor taunted her that unless she paid more she could expect other disasters to follow. Some other sects devised even more ingenious methods, including one that invented a graduated system of offerings. It was much like the awarding of college degrees. Depending on the amount, donations were classified, as first, second, pass and fail categories. Those who paid more were showered with eloquent lengthy prayers and the intensity and length of blessings would fade downwards. Those in the "fail" category would be treated to such rude stares that they would never wish to be found in that number again. As for AIDS patients staring death in the face, there was just no other category where they aspired to be rather than "first", even if it cost them the last of their earthly possessions.

Some religious sects falsely claimed that they possessed the powers to cure AIDS through prayer. Some uninfected people would be paraded as miraculously-cured AIDS patients. Fake laboratory results would be presented as evidence of the miracle to credulous and desperate people. For this and other reasons, some voluntary HIV/AIDS organisations in Uganda decided not to give out written AIDS results to clients, for fear that they could be misused. Also, a negative test today is not necessarily still negative three months later.

As AIDS bit harder many more opportunistic sects mushroomed and flourished. Inevitably the competition stiffened, and new innovative ways to entice clients were invented. Hurriedly constructed cheap churches, built using papyrus, known locally as Biwempe Churches, with even more powerful loudspeakers dubbed 'biwempe blasters" which kept the neighbourhood in a frustrated state of sleeplessness, sprang up everywhere so as to target the lucrative business. In fact, the old church song, *"Nearer my God to thee"*, would take on a new meaning, since a patient's death would likely be accelerated as less money was available for supportive medicines and nutritious food. The net effect to an individual AIDS patient was to make absolutely sure that at the end of it all, the usual funeral religious chant, *"I came with nothing in this world, and I leave with nothing"*, would be absolutely pertinent, down to the widow or widower and orphans left behind in utter poverty.

Even much later when AIDS therapy became more accessible, I was flabbergasted to see some patients abandon the life-saving therapy and die horribly, simply because some pseudo-pastors, after whatever money they had, convinced them that taking the treatment was tantamount to "lack of faith in the healing power of the Lord."

The Turning Point

It was hailed as the greatest news, to reach doomed AIDS patients and all the despairing AIDS care providers all over the world. To science it promised to be one of the greatest medical discoveries of all time. It was the turning point with regard to AIDS treatment and even seemed destined to do what was until then considered impossible. It all started happening in 1995, following the discovery of a new class of AIDS drugs known as Protease Inhibitors or PIs, as they later came to be abbreviated. The excitement in the medical and scientific community was palpable. New heroes, including Roy Gulick of New York University, were instantly created and became instant celebrities in medical circles. Gulick was one of the first researchers to supervise a study that confirmed the efficacy of a three drug combination AIDS treatment (triple therapy), consisting of a new drug called Indinavir, one of the newly discovered PI class of drugs, combined with two of the already known anti-AIDS drugs named Lamuvudine and Zidovudine. He tested the therapy on a cohort of ninety-seven patients with AIDS. The results were just incredible! As early as six months in the trial, it was abundantly clear that a revolution in HIV treatment was unfolding, and exciting scientific history was in the making.

Intrigued by the great news, I voraciously read everything about the evolving new drugs and learned as much as I could from my more up-to-date colleagues in the USA. The following year I attended the international AIDS conference that was held in Vancouver, Canada, where the stirring data were presented. I listened elatedly to the presentations. As I listened, I found myself wondering when and how I could quickly get hold of the new therapy for our people.

Unlike the then existing treatment regimen, the new therapy did not merely seem to postpone death but for the very first time promised a credible potential cure! Even the die-hard sceptics acknowledged that at the very least it restored hope that HIV could after all be tamed and be turned from a relentless killer into a treatable disease. Undeniably the hope and excitement was fully justified. There were vivid reports of very sick patients, including some on their death beds, who were being restored to health by the new therapy as their friends, relatives and doctors looked on in total amazement. To capture the dramatic health turn around, a graphic term *Lazarus Syndrome*, based on Lazarus who was raised from the grave by Jesus after being pronounced dead, was later coined to describe this phenomenon.

The key behind the landmark scientific breakthrough in the discovery of the new AIDS drugs was the advance in HIV molecular research, which shed light on the critical secrets of HIV proliferation in the human body. This resulted in much better understanding of the HIV physiology, especially its replication process and identification of the vulnerable stages at which it could be jammed or incapacitated by drugs. It was already known that the prime target of HIV is the vitally important CD4 cell, which plays a critical immunological role in protection against infections. The CD4 cells are recognisable to HIV because they have unique receptor sites to which the HIV bonds. Unlike most other viruses, which are made of DNA, HIV is an RNA variant. In its natural RNA form, HIV is unable to enter the core of the cell, which it must do, in order to replicate. To go around this obstacle, an enzyme called Reverse Transcriptase facilitates the transformation from the natural RNA-HIV into a DNA type, which enables it to enter the cell nucleus. Once inside, it then hijacks the cell resources, nourishes itself, and then goes on to replicate. Until 1995, the only available AIDS drugs, like AZT, targeted and incapacitated this crucial enzyme - Reverse Transcriptase. However, the agile HIV would find a way to go around this block mainly by mutation. This was the main reason why AZT by itself could not succeed in the treatment of AIDS. The new research revealed that the last stages of HIV replication required another key enzyme known as *protease* in order to complete the maturation stage, otherwise the reproductive circle is aborted. A new class of drugs known as *Protease Inhibitors* were developed to target this vital enzyme, and block the generation of new HIV virus. The combined effect of multiple drugs made it more difficult for the highly evasive virus to escape and develop resistance to the drugs. Doctors Gulick, Ho, Markowitz and other researchers demonstrated the power of combining three drugs that targeted these two crucial enzymes on HIV infection.

Plainly there was light at the end of the tunnel, and that development captivated the July 1996 Vancouver International AIDS Conference on AIDS and turned it into a triumphant celebration of victory of science over AIDS. This euphoria was most resonant in the rich Western countries, but must have reached a crescendo in the corridors of pharmaceutical companies that were poised to make a fortune. On the contrary there was only bemusement and muted curiosity in poor countries which, ironically with 90% of the disease burden should have had more cause for celebration. The killjoy was the price tag of US$14,000 per annum per patient. With over 11 million then estimated to be infected with HIV in Africa, simple arithmetic would demonstrate the unfeasibility of the new treatment. Evidently mass therapy for the poor was not even talked about, as it was just not plausible at least in the foreseeable future.

The issue of the moral imperative with regard to the deplorable AIDS catastrophe in Sub-Saharan Africa was just set aside. Obviously at the Vancouver AIDS conference, not many wanted to spoil the party with such sentiments. It was almost rude to ask. If one insisted, as I did, he or she would be shrugged off. In the midst of this anticipation, and at the time when scientific history was being made, poor countries, including Uganda, whose sections of populations were in danger of being wiped out by AIDS, were clearly on the outside looking in. The message to the poor countries was either that of indifference or open discouragement - just in case the Africans got carried away with ideas of introducing the highly sophisticated designer drugs to their miserable set up. These high priced drugs were not meant for them. The Vancouver conference was bombarded with presentations detailing highly sophisticated state of the art tests essential for safe and effective use of the new treatment. The exorbitant cost of the tests, added a couple of thousand dollars to the overpriced drugs, not to mention the required technical skills that seemed to put the new therapy beyond the means and necessary technical competence of poor countries.

The *Viral load,* test unlike the then well established CD4 test seemed to give a better scientific indication of the effectiveness of the new therapy, as well as better prediction of disease progression and survival. It measures the numbers of viral RNA copies per millilitre of blood using a technique known as Polymerase Chain Reaction (PCR). CD4, on the other hand, was only good for determination of the immunological stage of the disease and the prediction of the likelihood of some opportunistic infections. To make the concept of the new tests well understood, especially by non-scientists, we were shown vivid illustrations using the train model. Viral Load was compared to the speed of the train, indicating that the higher the speed the more the disease progression. CD4, on the other hand, were compared to the stations on the way to the final destination-a washed-away bridge ahead (unknown to the driver) symbolising death. Every station on the way indicated the closeness to apocalypse. The problem was that the two complimentary tests, which were to be established as routine and essential for optimum management of AIDS patients on HAART in the West, were just prohibitively expensive and technologically challenging for routine use in poor developing countries. It was said at the time that the challenges associated with the two tests in developing countries were almost insurmountable.

At the July 1996 Vancouver International AIDS conference, scientists explained the absolute precision timing that the new drugs' dosaging required, pointing out that this was beyond the competence of most African patients. Alarm clocks were recommended to patients in the West who had to wake up at the precise time during the night to take their doses. "The Africans have no watches and most of them use the sun to estimate the time! I shudder to think what would happen on a rainy day!" one delegate commented during discussions.

Then there was the incredible pill burden, which in some cases required patients to take up to twenty pills per day. Much was said about the poor hygiene in the African set up and especially the scarcity of clean water, which would make it virtually impossible for Africans to benefit from the new therapy. Up to now there are some funding agencies who give preference to clean water supply to AIDS patients in preference to life-saving ART drugs.

Over and above the many so-called "insurmountable constraints" there was the issue of some AIDS drugs that required refrigeration. "These drugs would just melt away in the African heat", alarmists proclaimed. Moreover, to add to the problems, the issue of drug toxicity arose. There was need for sophisticated laboratory monitoring of patients on the new therapy.

All these issues were carefully presented and illustrated at the AIDS conference with snapshots of the dire conditions pertaining to specially selected areas of Africa, aimed at driving the point home. To underscore the perceived infeasibility of the new drugs in Africa, some apologists expressed the view that it was just nobody's fault that Africa was in such an awful state. It looked like it would never be possible for Africa to ever use the state-of-the-art AIDS drugs. "Awfully sorry," was the usual expression, "but nothing could be done for the hapless Africans." The only option for Africa was to concentrate on prevention and supportive therapy, especially prophylaxis for opportunistic infections using the cheap Cotrimoxazole abundantly available in many parts of the Dark Continent. This was the core message that many Africans delegates took home from Vancouver, although many also took with them the glossy handouts profiling the new products provided free by the pharmaceutical companies.

In hindsight, it appears to me that the sophistication associated with use of these drugs was grossly exaggerated, and I heard that was deliberately so. The high technological skills and operation of the latest equipment, that were made to look like rocket science, were deliberately projected as virtually impossible in Africa. To top it off, one misguided sadist put it more crudely,

> If AIDS treatment was a glass of clean water, Africa would not afford it.

I recall a presentation in which one of the speakers praised the virtues of one poor African patient that he described as having demonstrated "great heroism" by dying gracefully, without clamouring for therapy. In essence poor African AIDS patients were to be really good boys and girls, and accept their fate quietly and gracefully. Anyway, there seemed just no alternative. Some African doctors left Canada with no other option but to encourage their patients to do just that.

I still have lingering memories of the captivating events of that memorable Vancouver AIDS international conference. It was the most scientifically significant AIDS conference as far as AIDS treatment breakthrough was concerned. I still see images of overflowing conference halls, as the newly found celebrity heroes of science presented mind-boggling scientific data. If one was late by just a few minutes for the sessions, it was standing room only. I vividly recall the mesmerising talk about tens of billions of HIV viruses being produced daily in a single infected individual and the rate at which the new drugs were able to reverse these breathtaking rates of multiplication. I recall one incredible mathematical model that David Ho presented, projecting a timetable for total elimination of the virus from the body. It was the highlight of the conference. One could have heard himself think as attentive participants listened to the incredible prospect of an imminent AIDS cure! some presenters even talked of new tests like lymph node biopsy to determine the "cure stage." The lymph nodes were some of the sanctuaries of HIV and if it was determined that the new treatment had successfully eliminated the virus from these hard-to-reach sites, then treatment would be stopped at that stage and the patient declared cured. I was interviewed on a local TV channel and I expressed my optimism that the new therapy would make a great difference in AIDS treatment. I called for the new therapy to be made accessible to our AIDS battered countries. The pace of it all was just like a dream. The prospect of a cure was all too good to be true - and that's exactly how it eventually turned out to be.

Although many theories and projections turned out to be grossly wrong, not all was lost. In fact the heroes were not at all discredited. On the contrary they had all contributed to what was to become a new and exciting era of effective AIDS treatment. The result was the birth of a new standard of care involving the newly dubbed Highly Active Anti-Retroviral Therapy or HAART. HAART converted the previously terminal killer disease into a controllable chronic illness. But as far as the AIDS ridden poor countries were concerned, the prohibitively expensive therapy was to remain as good as non-existent for almost a decade.

As I prepared to depart from Vancouver, I never accepted the notion that the new therapy was impossible to use in Africa. In fact, I left more determined than ever before to make it available in Uganda. However, it was still painful to acknowledge that without funding support the new therapy would be for only a tiny rich minority who would benefit while the vast majority of patients died not just of AIDS but of poverty. Not only did I go on to introduce the new therapy to Uganda but my centre also started carrying out the then state-of-the-art Viral Load tests in addition to the already well-established CD4 that were at the time said to be just impossible in Africa. My centre went on to become successful in the use of HAART; in the process, it saved thousands of lives which would otherwise have perished, just like the millions of other Africans who died while shamelessly the world had hit on a highly effective remedy that could have kept the vast majority of them alive and well. However, to get to this stage I had to overcome incredible challenges, including a narrow escape from imprisonment.

3

AIDS Dilemmas

AIDS and Prejudice

AIDS! The scary word that turned out to be the world's most easily recognised acronym was coined by the American Centre for Disease Control in 1982. It stands for Acquired Immune Deficiency Syndrome, a descriptive name that was given to the creepy disease that had broken out among the mainly white male homosexuals in America. As all the infected people died, AIDS came to symbolise impending death – and grisly suffering before the inevitable doom. As soon as AIDS was linked to homosexuality, it immediately became a dirty word, kicking off a worldwide AIDS stigma.

The initial term coined for the mysterious new disease in America was *"Gay Plague."* However, there was no hint of racism at the time.

In US, as everyone who was not gay was beginning to feel safe and secure, cases of AIDS started cropping up among the "straight" men, the heterosexuals. In fact, the very first men who were found to have AIDS and declaring that they were not gay were accused of lying. However, their accusers had to desist when women too started succumbing to the disease. It soon emerged that this new group of heterosexual victims were predominantly blacks of Haitian origin. With the realisation that blacks were involved, racism began to emerge. Initially the numbers of blacks involved were still relatively small. When AIDS was later confirmed in Africa and started spreading on a massive scale, then AIDS racism was truly born and has been on the rise ever since. Subsequently the AIDS epicentre was reallocated from its apparent birth place, the USA where it was first recognised, to Africa where it was fuelled by dire circumstances and augmented by rampant poverty, causing unprecedented devastation.

In the meantime, the powerful gay lobby in the US launched a highly effective prevention drive in the 1980s that included use of the "rubber" (the condom), and when antiretroviral drugs became available in mid-1990s, the gays in the US, unlike the Africans, had the wherewithal to quickly access them. This was followed by a sharp decline in the death rates in USA. The new AIDS trend in the US then shifted from the mainly well-to-do white gays to the lesser privileged African Americans and other minorities. However, to poor Africa the nightmare was just beginning. AIDS has so devastated Africa and become identified with it so much that now very few people still remember that AIDS' very first epicentre was in the USA.

Far from its first enclave in the USA, where it first affected mainly white people, AIDS had in no time unfolded into Africa's most devastating disaster. However, it was not readily apparent how two continents thousands of miles apart acquired the same disease. Some people, including explicit and circumlocutory racists, all kinds of weird assumptions but, increasingly, the unproven theory that HIV started off in Africa became predominant. The Africans, the world's most racially abused race, complained that all kinds of calamities are blamed on Africa for no other apparent reason other than racism. It was self evident that the raging debate about the origin of AIDS was initially based more on prejudice and speculation than facts.

Then a search for its origin intensified in Africa. The efforts were rewarded with the identification of Simian Immunodeficiency Virus (SIV) which was discovered among apes in the African forests. SIV was enthusiastically described as an erstwhile relative of HIV. To some people, that was the smoking gun they had been looking for. However, some black people both in Africa and America, reacting against age-old racism and realising that the disease predominantly affected their community, became suspicious of a conspiracy being played out here. To date, there are many who still strongly believe in this hypothesis. I have met some people who insist that the likelihood should not just be ruled out merely for lack of evidence - as it may just be dummy evidence deliberately planted to mislead. The burden of proof they insist should be put on the other side to prove that no conspiracy actually took place. However, even this would not be enough. There are others who believe in a scientific accident theory, an undercover experiment or programme that went awfully wrong!

On June 18, 2006, I was confronted with this school of thought during a discussion about AIDS and racism with the local community living around a black community high school, George Westinghouse High School, in a deprived area of Pittsburgh, USA. Some of them believed that HIV resulted from a well-planned and executed conspiracy followed by a high level ingenious cover-up. The depth of the feelings some community members felt and expressed about this complex issue were passionate and emotional.

"If it's not true, well and good" one middle aged lady said to me, "but if as seems likely there is someone out there responsible for this heinous crime then he must not be allowed to escape unpunished." she added.

Some of the questions that rose from the black community during the meeting included the following concerns:

> Why is it the black people being blamed? Why are Africans being held responsible for spreading the disease to America? We hear of such huge numbers of Africans dying: are there folks left out there?

An American white scientist, who strongly believes that HIV was brought to America from Africa, shared the platform with me at the meeting. He was asked to explain how HIV moved from Africa to USA. He had just one word brusque confident answer: "Aeroplane!" He did not bother with the small details, like the airport of departure, flight number, departure time and arrival time of the HIV export from Africa to America. Yet without this information or strong circumstantial scientific evidence, it just means that the "aeroplane" answer was at the very best just an educated guess. The silver lining, perhaps, was that this was the one "black" disease that did not go to America on the cramped slave ships. One such disease that did was Sickle Cell Anaemia, but this one is inherited almost exclusively by black people. We can therefore confidently prove that it did not travel on the "Mayflower". As HIV can be carried by anyone irrespective of race, the planes that presumably took it to America could just as well have taken it the other way since they fly in either direction.

However, talking personally to this pleasant scientist, whom I got to like and respect, I could see that he passionately believed that his conclusions were derived purely scientifically, and have not been disproved yet. Without a doubt, he would take strong exception to any suggestion that his conclusions had any racist connotation. He was in fact demonstrably very respectful of the black community's sensitivities and took care to address their concerns. I personally never saw any xenophobic tendency in him. However, opportunistic racists would have no quarrel with his conclusions. Apparently the basis for his very confident conclusion was that the apes which were identified as harbouring a virus with a similarity to HIV were identified in Africa. When some genetic similarities between HIV and Simian Immunodeficiency Virus (SIV), found in chimpanzees and monkeys in central and western parts of Africa, were identified it caught the imaginations of scientists and non-scientists alike, trying to figure out how SIV mutated to cause the human form of the disease. Numerous amazing theories, some of them absurd but none conclusively proven, were floated. The numerous theories put forward ranged from speculations that HIV could have been transmitted in contaminated polio vaccines used extensively in central Africa in the 1950s, to outright racist vulgar suggestions that some Africans got it from having sex with apes. Other presumptions floated included the so called "hunter theory" where apes blood contaminated the African hunters in the process of butchering them for food. All in all, the predominant theory was that the Africans somehow got the disease from apes and then passed it on to other races.

It has, however, been demonstrated that some genetic correlations between HIV and SIV are quite strong. There is indeed a distinct possibility, though not conclusively proven, that HIV mutated from apes indigenous to Africa, and there are various hypotheses as to how this may have come about, including the so called "Serial Passage" theory, which are beyond the scope of this book. However, this does not necessarily imply, that Africans got the disease first from apes and spread it all over the world. Since the explorations of Christopher Columbus, monkeys and other apes have been ferried out of Africa to many parts of the world. Because of the close proximity with Africa, Europe started importing apes much earlier. As far as medical research and especially pharmaceutical drugs development are concerned, apes have been used and sometimes abused extensively as the guinea pigs clearing experimental drugs for use or tests in man. Apes' blood and tissues have been used widely to culture some special medical bugs that cause human diseases, and in vaccines development. Even some scientists have considered use of apes' vital organs for human transplants. All this work has been done almost exclusively in the West. It is not only for research that apes were imported to the West. Apes are also commonly found in zoos, circuses, in homes as pets, and these are kept in much closer proximity to humans than wild apes in Africa. Even some apes of African origin are at large in the Americas.

There is a recent example in the 1960s where laboratory staff in Europe, who handled apparently healthy monkeys imported from Central Africa, suddenly fell sick and died from a mysterious disease. It was later found that the monkeys had infected them with the then unknown killer virus that was named Marburg, after the city in Germany where it was identified. The origin of the monkeys that transmitted the killer virus was the Democratic Republic of Congo, and they were flown out of Entebbe Airport in Uganda to Germany. As far as is known no Ugandans who loaded the deadly cargo at Entebbe, the Germans who downloaded them or those who captured the apes from the forests of Congo, died or even fell sick. One possible explanation is that they may not have been exposed to the monkeys as much as were the laboratory workers in Germany, or that they were only exposed in a way that did not allow the virus to be transmitted. If this lethal virus related to Ebola had been a slow one like HIV, the connection would not have been so easy to make. The workers would have continued living their normal lives and by the time the symptoms showed up seven to ten years later, the seeds of the epidemic would have been cast far and wide and the connection with the monkeys obscure. If it had resulted in an epidemic, the molecular finger printing would have shown that the virus was related to Ebola, and Africans would have been blamed for spreading it. Keeping such a scenario in mind, it is possible that the transformation (mutation) from SIV to HIV could have taken place anywhere, even if the apes had an African connection. It is also possible that the hunter is much less likely to be as extensively exposed to the raw monkey tissues and fluids than scientists who meticulously dissect the animals for experimental purposes in the West, or those that have contact with them on a day-to-day basis as pets.

As HIV seemed to break out in America and Africa at almost the same time, it is more scientific to keep an open mind while research continues. However, the intercontinental movement of people over the ages, other than slavery, has been overwhelmingly from the West to Africa in the form of colonialists, soldiers, tourists and expatriates. Therefore, the possibility that AIDS evolved in the West and was brought to Africa should be investigated further. The current research emphasis is lopsided, as it appears to concentrate on looking for evidence to support a preconceived theory, instead of null hypothesis that allows unbiased investigation. In Africa, especially Rakai, where AIDS was first confirmed in Uganda, the possibility that it was introduced into the area from outside is very much more likely than local evolution of the disease.

Where Africans are concerned prejudice is never far from the surface. However, it would be naïve to accuse everyone who thinks that AIDS evolved in Africa of racism, because there are some conceivable reasons to base such suspicions on. Topmost are the dire conditions on the continent that provide a fertile ground for infectious diseases. No wonder, HIV just spread like wild fire in Africa, and has not yet finished with the continent. Infectious diseases like and thrive in overcrowded areas with poor or no sanitation, where water is scarce or not protected, where there is chaos, and hunger, and where health and social service are poor. Africa (which the "Economist" magazine on its cover page once described as "the hopeless continent") is to some extent guilty of many of these unflattering attributes. As explained earlier, behind all this, the underlying cause of it all is poverty. Not race. However, such dismal conditions, which are good for disseminating an infectious disease, are not necessarily as good at seeding it in a new location, or starting a worldwide pandemic. For instance, it is virtually impossible for a cholera-infected African to start an epidemic in Manhattan. Yet it would be possible for a Singapore SARS patient to start an epidemic in Soweto. Poverty and the black race are often wrongly confused with each other in terms of cause and effect. It also does not necessarily mean that every way in which dire circumstances could have fuelled the AIDS epidemic in Africa actually happened. In some cases, a few racists have simply picked on their favourite stereotypes of Africa out of the many possible adverse elements that admittedly exist in the world's poorest continent. They pick some examples and then blow them out of proportion, often without even presenting any semblance of evidence or credible investigation.

One way in which HIV and many other diseases like hepatitis spreads is through the contaminated needles used for injections. In the West and more recently in the former Eastern European countries where HIV/AIDS has taken hold, injecting drug addicts who share needles has been responsible for a relatively big number of infections. However, this mode of HIV transmission has played an insignificant role in the vast Africa HIV epidemic. Yet, some European scientists attributed a much higher share of HIV transmission in Africa to needle contamination than the evident reality on the ground. They talked of dire African conditions, the rural mainly illiterate communities having no means or awareness to use disposable syringes, and therefore re-using syringes, without sterilising them. Then there were the mass immunisation programmes for childhood infections, and pregnant women being exposed to contaminated needles during antenatal visits or delivery being blamed for the spread. It was stated that contaminated needles account for many AIDS cases, especially those that do not seem to fit the traditional modes of transmission. Certainly contaminated needles are not mainly responsible for the pandemic explosion in Africa. If contaminated injections were to blame for a high percentage of transmissions, then African children and the elderly would have a higher HIV prevalence than they actually do because they would be expected to receive even more injections than the healthier sixteen to forty-five year olds.

All data across Africa indicate that the high-risk groups for HIV do not necessarily coincide with those that were exposed to potentially-contaminated injections. One would have just ignored this theory, but it is such publications that make news headlines. Indeed this proved to be the case. Such controversial reports were disseminated so widely in the mass media that the World Health Organisation and some care providers in Africa worried about possible negative consequences for HIV preventive programmes. In Africa, however, where millions of people were already infected, where the disease was still spreading like wildfire, and where there were no resources to purchase the exorbitant HIV treatment or drugs for prevention of mother to child transmission (PMTCT), this was a potentially very dangerous development because it would convey a wrong message. Africa's only hope was a robust preventive programme that targeted and prioritised the real factors responsible for the runaway scourge. The place of contaminated needles in the priority hierarchy was towards the bottom of the list, and was already being given due attention in all preventive programmes. However, diverting scarce resources from priority areas would have cost many more lives.

Therefore, I was happy to join other scientists in writing a rebuttal letter, to explain that the role of contaminated needles in the spread of HIV in Africa should not be unduly exaggerated. We warned against abandoning priority life-saving preventive measures which could have possibly arisen as a result. However, we emphasised the role of safer disposable syringes as part of the strategies of HIV prevention. There are, of course, some other reasons for concerns about the injection theory but it is not necessary to go in details, since there is irrefutable evidence to demonstrate that it is heterosexual sex that by far drove the AIDS epidemic in Africa. This is followed by mother to child transmission, while other factors, including blood transfusions and contaminated needles, played a relatively small role.

Talking of heterosexual sex as the main route of HIV transmission in Africa tunes another set of racists' imaginations into top gear: "Look ,Africans are doing it anywhere with anyone, any time and every time, getting themselves finished by AIDS in the process." Serious studies exploring the sexual practices of different races have found more myths than surprises. African sexuality is no different from that of other races. It is the other special risk factors led by poverty that make Africans vulnerable, not their skin colour. For instance, the fastest growing AIDS epidemic is now in Eastern Europe and Asia. Eastern Europe, including the former world superpower Russia, Rumania, Bulgaria and others, have recently been hard hit by AIDS following the collapse of communism. The sudden shift from a socialist economy to capitalism left many families that used to depend on state subsides in abject poverty. Many of them live in dire conditions that sometimes look worse than those in some African countries. Not unlike Zimbabweans, many of their citizens have been on the move mainly as economic refugees in Europe and even as far away as Dubai. Russian prostitutes in Dubai are reportedly doing brisk business, and some rackets of underground gangs are minting money from illegal smuggling of young Eastern European girls to Western Europe for prostitution. Meanwhile the huge populations of Asia are masking the huge number of HIV-infected people. Everywhere, the epidemic is especially marked among the poor living in conditions not dissimilar to Africa, or worse.

While these tragic events were unfolding in Africa, in America the AIDS epidemic was quickly transforming from being a disease of mainly well-to-do white homosexuals to relatively poor immigrant Haitians, and African-Americans. The HIV rates also went up in other minorities,especially the Latino communities, and eventually surpassed that of the white communities. Currently, the African-Americans in proportion to the size of their population now dominate the epidemic in the US. The shift in the epidemic's dynamics was driven by the same factor as in Africa, Eastern Europe and Asia, namely poverty. These days in USA we do not hear so much of rich people of the likes of the late Rock Hudson and Michael Jordan. It is now the poor, who do not usually get media attention, that are the new face of AIDS. The same scenario pertains in Europe. In almost all major Western European cities proportionally more blacks per population have AIDS than the whites. Some AIDS clinics in London are almost exclusively patronised by Africans.

With regard to the contrasting effects of poverty, race and AIDS, the situation in South Africa, with the biggest white community in Africa, provides a good illustration. The South African blacks are overwhelmingly infected by HIV as compared to their white counterparts even when the population ratios are taken into account. Also, the rate at which HIV/AIDS swept across South Africa is just breathtaking even by African standards. Aside from race, these two communities could be mistaken as living in two different worlds. Most white South Africans because of apartheid ensured a standard of living most Europeans in Europe just dreamed about. Meanwhile the black majority were because of racist laws condemned to inhumane treatment under legislation that was calculated to ensure perpetual servitude and poverty. A visitor to South Africa does not need any guide to determine where the different races live. If you come to a big house, in a good location with well-kept lawns, a swimming pool and uniformed black armed guards opening the gate for a uniformed black maid, then you just know that the people living there are white. If, on the other hand, you come to a filthy slum area full of what are called in the South African jargon, matchbox houses, in numbered rows (designed more for ease of access of apartheid police than comfort) in deprived areas, that is where black people live and where AIDS is found.

The fact that AIDS has taken on a black hue has not gone unnoticed by racists, who have not bothered to find out the real reasons behind it all or, if they somehow stumbled on it, just ignored it. Almost everywhere you find substantial black populations, you can take "YES" for an answer even before you ask whether there is AIDS in that community. That is smoking gun enough for any racist. However, discrimination against Africans is not only in AIDS. It is to blame for some of the conditions that nurture many other disasters, and the explanation for the almost always poor, late, too little or just no responses to virtually all calamities that befall Africa or peoples of African origin living anywhere in the

Diaspora. A very recent example of discrimination against blacks in the Diaspora was the shocking televised footage of mainly black people in distress when the colourful city of New Orleans in USA was devastated by hurricane Katrina in the last week of August 2005. By August, 30, 80% of the city was underwater. From Africa the poorest continent in the world, we watched in total disbelief as mainly black survivors of the disaster were denied emergency aid by the richest country on earth - leaving them to suffer horrific conditions, just like most poor victims of calamities in Africa. As devastation overwhelmed the city, the bodies of those who could not flee, mainly because of poverty, floated in the flood waters along what had a couple of weeks earlier been bustling streets and lively jazz entertainment joints. Proportionally more of the bodies were Black. As flood levels rose higher and higher, people trapped in their houses ended up taking refuge on the roofs. The roofs was bleak and with mainly black people clinging on.

"Surely that can't be happening in America!" was a common exclamation. It was not the finest hour for America. In the immediate aftermath of the disaster, many were outraged by the shamefully slow response in alleviating the plight of the poor, especially the blacks. To underscore the desperation of the calamity, one anguished woman survivor, who was desperately looking for shelter, sorrowfully commented, "If we were lucky, we would have died." In response to the apparent failure to rush in and save mainly black people the *CBS Radio News* quoted the New Orleans City Councilman, Oliver Thomas, saying that, "People are too afraid of black people to go in and save them." However, some people insisted that racism was not a factor and that it was poor people in general who were affected and not specifically blacks. In response, Rev Jesse Jackson said that race was "at least a factor" and added, "We have an amazing tolerance for black pain!"

In terms of sheer numbers of lives lost in past disasters, including genocides, absolutely nothing exceeds the devastation caused to Africans by the denial of life-saving AIDS drugs. As discussed elsewhere, this was the saddest epoch for humanity. As Africans in their millions died a painfully slow death, the drugs were where the money was, but not where the disease was. The rich countries had it within their powers to intervene and put a stop to the devastation of Africans, but did not. All concerned in this debacle would vehemently deny any racist motives, and would instead blame the "rampant chronic unsolvable African problems" that were beyond the control of anyone. Nobody denies that Africans like any other race have their share of blame and are responsible for some of the dismal conditions that have wreaked havoc on their own kith and kin, especially through bad leadership. Never mind that leaders like Amin and Mobutu would not have taken over power without the support of the West. Even when this is taken into account, callous inaction in the face of such disaster cannot be justified. It is sad that the ugly face of prejudice kept peeping through in this truly human tragedy.

However, the worst form of discrimination and the most common in HIV/AIDS is not the overt old-fashioned kind which is no longer politically acceptable. In the modern era, the old-fashioned discrimination is much less dangerous because it can be easily spotted and fought, and suffered less painfully than the veiled form. This is because one would never knows when the concealed variety hits you. Sometimes you do not even know whether you are a victim of it or not, and this is more so if it is shrouded in a legitimate process like a bureaucratic procedure, or a legal process like the amazing events described in the next chapter. This situation comes about because in the performance of many public duties there is always some leeway for individuals to exercise a degree of self-regulating judgement. If one reached a decision based on a racially-prejudiced motive, it would (unless it is overt) be inadvertently protected by law. Sometimes discrimination is by proxy. For instance, in apartheid South Africa some white racists used blacks to implement their intolerant agenda against other blacks. With regard to HIV/AIDS too, I have seen some instances where unsuspecting people living with HIV/AIDS have been used by opportunists to advance their agenda usually by discrediting people or organisations not toeing their line. At the international level, patents laws, TRIPS and WTO are on paper non-racist but just check on the colour of the majority of the people who suffer as a result of their decisions.

Discrimination is bad enough without AIDS, but much worse with it. Yet AIDS has absolutely no respect for race or geographical borders. It just targets and victimises any susceptible humans, especially the poor – because poverty and not race makes them especially susceptible. Prejudice regarding AIDS directly and indirectly contributed in making a very awful situation truly catastrophic.

The Death Sentence

The gruesome television footage of corpses of African illegal immigrants to Europe floating in the Mediterranean, and the bodies of those shot trying to climb over the cages erected in some European refugee reception areas to keep the Africans out, underscores the scope of desperation brought about by poverty and the predicament faced by many Africans trying to escape it. Against all odds, some refugees make it to the rich West hoping for a better life. Those that make it have come to be known as economic refugees. But it is only a tiny minority that achieves success in Europe. Even in their new home they remain at the bottom of society facing formidable obstacles. However, from the mid-1990s, Europe started receiving a new category of much more desperate and undesirable refugees. These were AIDS refugees. They went in a daring last gamble to escape the death sentence that AIDS without access to the life-saving antiretroviral drugs meant to them.

The natural humanitarian response to a catastrophic emergency of this magnitude would have been an immediate international mobilisation to rush the life-saving therapy to the anguished Africans in Africa. As many health care providers as possible, including volunteers, would have been marshalled to help. However, as is often the case, the AIDS crisis inclusive, if Africa is on fire (for instance the apartheid atrocities in South Africa that were allowed to go on for far too long, the Rwanda genocide that killed hundreds of thousands before any international intervention, or more recently the crisis in Darfur region of Sudan), no one seems to be in a hurry to put out the flames. The few organisations that move at a snail's pace into Africa to help put out the fires tend to pull in when it is too late, or come in poorly equipped with only a few buckets of water instead of fire engines. Nonetheless, the few buckets are too often publicised with great trumpet blast and the results too wildly exaggerated. But almost always you never fail to hear a coded phrase "considering the dire circumstances" added, to explain the inevitable outcome in advance.

During the second half of 1990s and early 2000s, scores of Ugandans on AIDS treatment in the United Kingdom (UK) suffered a double jeopardy of AIDS and some astounding legal entanglements that were to consume a lot of my time as I worked with the British lawyers, doctors and humanitarian organisations to save their lives. Their horrendous ordeal started when some of them sought to legally extend their stay on the advice of their British doctors in order to continue the treatment they could not live without. It started in 1995, when a few letters started trickling in from British doctors worried about their Ugandan AIDS patients living in the UK. Apparently they needed my help - to provide collaborative medical evidence from Uganda to strengthen their submission to the immigration department in support of their patients' continued stay in Britain so that they could continue to benefit from the life-saving AIDS therapy they were providing them with. The doctors pleaded that if their patients were sent back to Uganda they would die because antiretroviral therapy and the monitoring tests would not be accessible to them. In the mid-1990s the AIDS patients were not many and my letters explaining that we had few resources and facilities to treat AIDS patients in Uganda were readily accepted and the patients allowed to stay. The UK immigration would not deport anyone unless it was shown that the concerned patient's life was not in danger.

However the situation changed suddenly after 1996 following the discovery of the truly-life saving AIDS treatment that was dubbed Highly Active Antiretroviral Therapy (HAART). The long craved-for news of its discovery got headline publicity all over the world. Within a short time it had become the standard care in the West resulting in a sharp decline in AIDS deaths. But it came with a price tag that put it beyond almost all Ugandans, with the exception of an insignificant minority. The only hope for survival was to seek treatment in Europe or America where the life-saving drugs were. However for all, except a few desperate patients, abject poverty put their dreams of escaping death by travelling abroad far beyond achievable reality. All that was offered to AIDS patients in Uganda was the general advice to "live positively." Therefore the numbers of Ugandan patients that successfully made it to the UK were not many. However, they were in the eyes of the British immigration department big enough to make them see red - actually black!

The British National Health Services (NHS) and their staff are some of the very best public health service providers in the world despite problems brought about by privatisation and under-funding. The service is also free if one qualifies or comes in as an emergency case. Naturally most sick Ugandan AIDS patients who went to the UK made a bee-line for the NHS for treatment as soon as they arrived. From the letters I received from the UK many of them arrived there when they were at death's door, and indeed some were admitted as emergency cases. Miraculously, almost all of them were saved from death, thanks to the power of modern ARVs and medical expertise. With a new lease of life, their health and strength restored, they now faced a dilemma: what next? Returning to Uganda was not an option for many of them, because the drugs they needed to take every day in order to remain healthy were not available. Yet staying in the UK was dogged with immigration problems, and those that stayed illegally risked arrest and deportation. In any case, AIDS infected men cannot live by the ARVs alone. They needed to find work and earn a living. That's when trouble started, and by 1998 many AIDS patients were in trouble. Scores of them frantically tried to regularise their stay by seeking *AIDS asylum* - which must have been a new term in the British Home Office jargon - while some others were rounded up and deported. Threatened with removal back to the spectre of death from which they had escaped and feared, many terrified Ugandan AIDS patients in the UK resorted to immigration lawyers, charity organisations and AIDS support groups for help.

Desperate AIDS patients with the backing of their doctors, humanitarian organisations and mainly charity lawyers, pleaded for them to be allowed to stay in the UK on the grounds that they would die, since the ARVs that kept them alive would not be accessible to them if they were sent back to Uganda. However, some elements within the immigration department seemed determined to get rid of them and went to extraordinary lengths to prove that the very same AIDS drugs were freely and widely available in Uganda. While "free" was just a blatant lie, it was true that a very small quantity of AIDS drugs was available at cost recovery price for the very few rich patients who could afford them. This was the true definition of "availability" in Uganda, which was meaningless to the vast majority of AIDS patients who died en masse because they could not afford them. It was like proving that there is gold in Timbuktut to the poor Moroccans. The two things ARVs had in common with gold were the price tag and inaccessibility to the poor. AIDS drugs were so exorbitantly priced that for all practical purposes they were as good as non-existent in Africa. The result was bloodbath in Sub-Saharan Africa. This was the chilly reception that awaited any poor AIDS deportee from London – a guaranteed slot on the AIDS slaughter chain. Thus their deportation would be tantamount to a death sentence - albeit by proxy.

From 1996, I was bombarded with frantic requests from doctors, lawyers and humanitarian organisations in the UK including the Terrence Higgins Trust, a pioneer HIV-AIDS charity, to come to the aid of many distressed Ugandan AIDS patients and help to save them from imminent expulsion. The letters that had started as a trickle had by the end of 1998 turned into a flood. The requests were so frequent and frantic that some days I would find myself more occupied with legal than my usual medical work. A few years later, the requests were overwhelming. At one time I tried writing a general all-encompassing letter to the numerous UK lawyers, and humanitarian organisations but it was swatted down by the immigration department that kept bouncing back with new evidence to justify throwing out Ugandan AIDS patients. The determination to remove the AIDS patients was so intense that they kept shifting the goalposts. Therefore I had no alternative but to keep addressing new questions, as they emerged. It was not that the immigration department had any difficulty in finding out the truth about the dire situation of AIDS in Uganda because the information was freely available. The gruesome pictures of AIDS carnage in Africa were not uncommon spoilers of British dinners as they were frequently aired on BBC television evening news and were also the subject of numerous prime time documentaries. Instead, the immigration department seemed to look for the kind of collaborators who would provide them with enough justification to help them to get rid of the unwanted AIDS patients. However, it is recognised that the immigration department has a responsibility to determine whom to allow in their country or reject. But British law protects the vulnerable. Accordingly, the immigration department had determined that they would not send away any AIDS patients already on life-saving therapy in UK unless they proved that the same treatment would be continued in their own country. So the blame for removing AIDS patients on false grounds would mostly be put on the shoulders of those that deliberately provided the false evidence.

The immigration department succeeded in getting incredibly murky evidence. It later transpired that this misleading information was being provided clandestinely to the immigration authorities from a then anonymous source in Uganda. Their nameless source had lied to them that AIDS drugs were freely available at the Joint Clinical Research Centre in Kampala and that Uganda was the best place in the world to be for anyone with AIDS! As I was at the time one of the very few doctors running a sizeable formal AIDS treatment clinic in Uganda, I was frequently asked by lawyers and doctors to write and explain the situation the deportees would face on their enforced homecoming. One typical letter read in part:

Bloomsbury, London, 22 January 1998

Dear Dr Mugyenyi

I am a solicitor instructed on behalf of a Ugandan family in which the mother and daughter are HIV positive. The British Immigration Service is trying to deport the mother and daughter from the UK and we have applied to the High court to challenge this deportation. … I would be grateful if you were able to deal with the queries contained in the attached letter. You will note from the letter that we have a first hearing date in Court on the 9th February 1998 and therefore need to gather information as a matter of urgency.

The queries that the lawyer referred to were whether antiretroviral drugs were available and free of charge in Uganda as alleged, and whether they were accessible through clinical trials. He also wanted to know also whether children under the age of six were acceptable into clinical trials. I found out later that the lawyer was trying to counter the lies of an immigration contact in Uganda whose evidence they were inadvertently trying to use to send back the poor child and her mother to the abyss. Apparently the British doctors were also involved in a fight to save the lives of their Ugandan AIDS patients. For instance, one of the doctors wrote the following letter of support to a lawyer representing his patient, which in part read:

> *...it is my unreserved opinion that it would be unreasonable and inadvisable to expect Ms X to go and live in Uganda ... Unfortunately there is a huge divide between (medical) management that can be offered here in the UK versus that which is available in a developing country such as Uganda. As far as I am aware neither ART nor essential laboratory monitoring procedures for CD4 and Viral Load would be available to Ms X should she move to live in Uganda. This would obviously impact greatly on her general well being and likely life expectancy. I would also point out that there would be other risks to her health if she lived in Africa such as tuberculosis, tropical diseases and water borne sources of gastrointestinal infections.*

The doctor's use of the term "likely life expectancy" was just a polite way of saying that she would die. However, this was a special case. The concerned lady was a British citizen. Her woes were due to the fact that she was married to a Ugandan man who was facing deportation and secondly she had AIDS. Normally spouses of British citizens would have been spared this threat. However, in this case which also involved AIDS, the rules were tightened, and the marriage connections were not very helpful. It was indeed true that a woman who had lived in the UK all her life and in addition had AIDS would be at increased risk of some tropical diseases like malaria.

Meanwhile, letters continued to pour in from organisations and from lawyers representing an increasing number of AIDS-infected Ugandans in various states of distress, and stages of deportation proceedings. I kept busy writing countless letters endlessly explaining the grim situation facing AIDS patients in Uganda. Indeed I was in a unique position to know the facts because in my capacity as the director of the pioneer AIDS treatment and research centre in Uganda, I was a firsthand witness to the nightmare. I patiently provided detailed descriptions of the gruesome fate that deportees would face. I described the AIDS carnage all around me that I witnessed almost on a daily basis. I emphasised that too many people had died and many more were dying needlessly, simply because they had no access to antiretroviral therapy. I explained that it was not that some drugs were not physically available in Uganda, because I had made sure that they were always available at the Joint Clinical Research Centre, but that they were unaffordable. Thus, the vast majority of Ugandan AIDS patients just perished, dying of a disease that had ceased to be a killer in the UK. This information was initially enough to allow the beleaguered Ugandans to stay. However, by the end of 1999, I noticed a sudden change. The conditions for Ugandans seeking AIDS asylum once more started getting harder and harder. The "magic wand" that my letters used to produce seemed to have waned. Once more the UK lawyers and doctors faced a tough time with the immigration service, as their Ugandans clients were once more threatened with deportation orders. Some were deported including one woman who arrived back with only three months drugs supply for a life-time disease!

"What's up?" I faxed the question to one of the lawyers that I had got to know over the years through frequent correspondences about the Ugandan cases. I wanted him to explain the flurry of letters that had resurged after a relative lull. However, before he could reply I got the answer from another lawyer also struggling to save yet another Ugandan family from deportation. It came as a copy of a deportation order written by the Immigration Department to a solicitor representing a Ugandan woman facing deportation. The revealing letter read:

Immigration and Nationality Directorate

Croydon 04/04/2000

Dear Sir

I refer to your application of 10/11/98 for further leave to remain in the UK. After careful consideration, it has been decided to refuse the application for the reasons stated on the refusal notice.

The Secretary of State has considered whether there are sufficient grounds to justify allowing your client to stay in the UK exceptionally, in particular her ill health. However, I have contacted the British High Commission in Kampala who have advised that some of the top HIV research teams in the world are in Uganda and the care and treatment of those with HIV is available.

Furthermore I understand that the CD4 counts, viral load and viral sensitivity are all done routinely as part of UNAIDS initiative, and that this research benefits thousands of Ugandans who are on triple therapy. In addition to this antiviral drugs are available through 4 public centres at remarkable subsidised prices in Uganda.

The Secretary of State is therefore not satisfied that should Mrs X have to return to her own country she would have no access to the medication that she needs. The Secretary of State therefore refuses your client's application ...

If your client does not wish to exercise a right of appeal against this decision, she should make arrangements to leave the UK within 28 days of the refusal notice.

Evidently the sudden changes in the fortunes of the Ugandan AIDS patients in Britain had emanated from the British High Commission in Kampala. The letter was very worrying because it contained false and misleading information. There was something else about this letter, however, that did not appear quite right to me. It was rather un-British. Right away I doubted that the usually well-informed British High Commission would have been so out of touch to this extent. Surely they knew better than this. Their Ugandan High Commission workers must have been dying like thousands of other Ugandans. Their local staff would have been absent from work countless times in order to attend funerals. They must have heard lamentations of Ugandan AIDS patients unable to access AIDS drugs. The local Kampala newspapers carried harrowing stories of AIDS patients in desperation on almost daily basis. Very sad stories of AIDS orphans and AIDS infected children in dire circumstances in Uganda must have been well known to the embassy. The embassy must have been bombarded with desperate requests for help with AIDS treatment. Surely the British High Commission in Uganda cannot have been an island in the midst of mayhem. Therefore, it did not make sense to me that this misinformation was the work of the High Commission. I still don't believe that it was. Yet quite clearly there was absolutely no reason that I could discern why the immigration office could not be believed. Certainly they did not just make up the story. Therefore it just looked to me that this was an individual or a rogue person within the High Commission who supplied the misleading information without necessarily passing it through official channels. The information supplied indicated that it came from someone with some basic medical knowledge but certainly not up to speed with the latest in HIV/AIDS medicine. I kept wondering who this "agent provocateur" could be. Fortunately I did not have to wait long for an answer. One of the lawyers whose client was the victim of the same misinformation had apparently managed to obtain a copy of the letter from the hitherto unknown source of misinformation in Kampala.

The lawyer wrote:

London 6 April 2000

I have seen many useful letters from you about the availability of treatment for HIV and AIDS in Uganda. I am a solicitor who used to work at a community legal centre. I am now in private practice, where I continue to work with Ugandan nationals living with HIV.

I am writing to ask for your assistance. I am dealing with a case at present where I have been provided with a letter from (one I call) Dr X dated 22nd October 1999. I enclose a copy. I am very concerned about its contents and was wondering whether you would be able to comment on each of his paragraphs and let me know whether you agree with the statements that he made. In addition it would be helpful if you could give me your views on the availability of free treatment for HIV and AIDS in Uganda.

This letter solved a mystery for me. The source of this new misery of the Ugandan AIDS sufferers in the UK and the new barrage of mails from solicitors was now clear. Unbelievably it was one expatriate Kampala-based doctor whom I knew quite well. I was dumbfounded by the extent to which this fellow was prepared to go, not excluding telling blatant lies, in order to have the AIDS infected Ugandans thrown out of the UK. Yet as a resident in Uganda, he knew very well the bleak situation they would face if they were returned to Uganda. Apparently he worked with an embassy contact who was very careful to blacken out his or her name on the letter before it was passed on to the immigration people in the UK. It was evidently meant to provide potent armaments to help deport AIDS infected Ugandans in the UK and dissuade anyone contemplating going to Britain for AIDS treatment. Never mind that most Ugandans AIDS patients were too poor to even make the road journey to Entebbe airport even if they got an express invitation to Britain! Dr X's damning letter is reproduced verbatim:

Kampala, 22 october1999

HIV and AIDS are very common in Uganda and the country has become the focus of many aid and research programmes. Some of the top virologists from CDC and MRC are working in Uganda. With 400,000 people with HIV and one of the best treatment and research programmes in the world, it is astonishing to read that treatment is not available and inconceivable to envisage 400,000 Ugandans going to UK or Europe for treatment when it is so much cheaper here in Uganda.

These are up to date facts.

We routinely do CD4 count and Viral Loads, and a new UNAIDS programme is enrolling 300 people for free viral load and viral drugs sensitivity tests 5 times a year as part of a new research programme.

Drugs are very widely available and very highly subsidised both by the manufacturers and by various agencies. Over 800 people are getting drugs at up to 50% less as part of one major programme alone! The enclosed price list is already out of date as more drugs have become available and prices have come down further. One of my patients on triple therapy using Combivir and Saquinivir had a bill this month of only 430$ from JCRC.

This week a patient of mine with a rising viral load was switched from AZT 3Tc and saquinivir to DDI, Stavudine and nevirapive after 2 samples were taken for free sensitivity testing 2 months apart. I wonder how many centres in Europe do viral sensitivity testing free?

Not surprising some of my European AIDS patients try to stay in Uganda to take advantage of this remarkable service, and I believe any Ugandan in Europe with HIV should return here as soon as possible to benefit from one of the best HIV research and treatment programmes in the world.

Incredible! This was the mole that provided misinformation to the Home Office. Apparently the immigration officer had just lifted Dr X's quotes with the language unchanged and used it in the letter to the lawyer and as a basis for rejecting the application of his client. I was outraged. But why was Dr X doing this? Dr X of all people knew the whole truth, about the carnage and dire circumstances AIDS patients faced in Uganda. Yet it was apparent that his letter was at the very best a ham-fisted attempt to help the immigration department get rid of the AIDS infected Ugandans irrespective of the consequences. At worst it was a xenophobic attitude he held deep in his heart for the Ugandan people he lived amongst. I immediately replied to the UK lawyer taking care to be as polite as possible, as follows:

10th April 2000

I am astonished by Dr X's letter, which generally project incorrect information about HIV situation in Uganda as well as availability of treatment.

While it is true that some research programmes are taking place in Uganda, it is important to note that CDC and MRC Research programmes are not health provision programmes as can be confirmed by the agencies concerned.

As is normal in all ethical medical research protocols, only volunteers receive some free tests and sometimes research treatment, which may include placebo (or blanks). There is currently no research project providing free antiretroviral combination therapy in Uganda.

It is false to state that there are only 400,000 people who are living with HIV in Uganda. The conservative estimate of the Ministry of Health states that at least 1.4 million people are living with AIDS in Uganda. It is extremely frustrating to read that "Uganda has one of the best treatment and research programmes in the world," when in fact the treatment situation is desperate for the poor patients in our resource constrained country! Try that statement on the thousands of AIDS patients who have no access to even the rudiments of HIV treatment!

Joint Clinical Research Centre pioneered routine screening and monitoring of HIV infection and treatment in Uganda, doing tests like CD4 and viral loads. Only those participating in some few ongoing funded research projects that require these tests as part of the protocol get them free. The rest of the patients have to pay for these tests. Needless to say only a tiny minority can afford the cost of these tests, leave alone the cost of antiretroviral drugs.

Antiretroviral drugs are available at an unaffordable cost in Uganda and I think in most other neighbouring countries as well, but there is hardly any subsidy to talk about. Only two pharmaceutical companies have joined the so-called access initiative, but even these have not made any impact on the cost. I enclose the current price list from UNAIDS supported non-profit company specifically set up to import anti HIV drugs for your update confirmation. There is no programme in Uganda which offers 50% discount on anti HIV drugs and the reported number of over 800 getting drugs at this cost is fictitious.

It is possible that Dr X's patients got drugs at a cost of US $450 from JCRC for a combination that includes Saquinavir. In the current recommendation for HIV treatment, Saquinavir old formulation hard gel capsules (the only ones available at JCRC) are no longer recommended. Its use is a desperate measure and we are soon abandoning it. Be that as it may, a bill of $450 per month is far and above the average salary of even the high professionals like hospital doctors and other graduate workers in Uganda's public service. Anti HIV drugs at the current cost are just not sustainable or available in Ugandan public hospitals for general use ...

As per last paragraph words just fail me when he states that:

" – any Ugandan in Europe with HIV should return immediately to benefit from one of the best HIV research and treatment programmes in the world"

It sounds to me like an invitation for patients to come and die at home. I presume this was written for people totally ignorant of the desperate nature in which HIV/AIDS patients live, not only in Uganda but throughout the Sub-Saharan Africa.

Indeed if there was any such available treatment programme in Uganda the country would be flooded with equally desperate patients from neighbouring countries whose conditions are similarly miserable.

Lastly I have talked to Dr X to express my personal concern over his writing. As the secretary to the Uganda AIDS drugs access initiative as well as director of one of the leading research centres on HIV/AIDS in Uganda, I am in position to know the basic facts concerning HIV situation in Uganda. You may contact other experts in the Ugandan Ministry of Health's AIDS control programme, UNAIDS in Geneva, or MRC based right next door in London who would confirm these facts.

I faxed the letter to the lawyer who rushed it to the immigration department to try and save his worried AIDS infected Ugandan clients from imminent deportation.

Nine days later I received the lawyers reply:

London 19 April 2000

Just a quick line to thank you so much for dealing so promptly and effectively with Dr X's letter. You will be pleased to hear that once I provided your letter to the Home Office they backed down and have conceded the case I have been dealing with.

I hope that you won't mind that I have copied your letter to the Terrence Higgins Trust for their library and use in similar cases.

Thank you so much for your help.

I was right to suspect that the information purported to have come from the British embassy to the Home Office was actually not an official embassy communication. It was just too shallow. However, it was now confirmed that Dr X was working with someone in the embassy, a sort of middleman whose job it was to pass on his letter to the Home Office. Whoever it was, he or she was not doing a "day time" kind of job. The fact that Dr X worked with such a person and obligingly went over board in his report is interesting. I found myself wondering: what sort of allegiance would a person like Dr X have to the people of Uganda - a country that had provided him a livelihood and a home? Was this the normal way to repay the desperately ill citizens of one's adopted country in need of life-saving medicine? Was he right to stand on a higher moral ground and judge and hurt poor people who were engaged in a desperate fight for their very lives, when he himself had moved to make a living in their country - not as a missionary or selfless community physician but as a general practitioner? That is assuming, of course, that he did not have another undeclared job. What drives such a person? What ever it is, it certainly did not exude any noticeable humanitarian scent.

Dr X himself soon re-confirmed that he worked with some individual in the British Embassy. Apparently the letter I wrote to the lawyer, a copy of which was in the hands of the Home Office, must have embarrassed his contact. His own letter was so obviously naïve with incredible statements like *"doing viral drugs sensitivity tests 5 times a year"* (nobody in the world needs such routine monitoring of AIDS patients) or *"Europeans trying to stay in Uganda in order to access AIDS treatment services."* Such overt expressions of ignorance must have raised the eyebrows of anyone who bothered to give it a second glance. No person with any basic information about the AIDS pandemic could have believed such a letter even without the benefit of knowing Uganda. Curiosity and disappointment led me to call Dr X on the phone to ask why he found it necessary to convey such wrong information. I drew a blank! However to his contact in the British embassy, he must have felt that he had to respond to my letter, and accordingly wrote a self-protective letter. However, this time round the name was not blackened out. In terms of the quality of the letter, it was even worse than the first one. It, demonstrated however, that Dr X was unapologetic and still resolute to fight AIDS infected Ugandans in the UK. His professed reasons for doing so were, however, very depressing.

In his letter dated July, 11,2000, in which he tried to undo the damage my letter must have caused to his credibility at the Home Office, he wrote to say that my letter had in fact confirmed all his points. His first justification of this strange statement was that my letter had confirmed the presence of AIDS expertise in Uganda, and he named me as being among them. Interestingly, he did not include himself among the experts yet there he was dishing out "expert opinions" on which peoples' lives depended. He did not bother to explain what good the presence of experts would do for the deportees on arrival if they could not provide them with the essential AIDS life saving drugs, or essential monitoring tests, for the simple reason that they were not affordable. Secondly, he picked on the estimated number of 1.4 million Ugandans living with HIV/AIDS, and ignored his own grossly underestimated numbers and said this confirmed his point that "it is not conceivable to send them all to UK for treatment." As his letter was being written to the British embassy, it is perhaps understandable that he included this alarmist statement presumably to arouse the fear of the UK being overwhelmed by marauding HIV-infected Ugandans! This also would perhaps help divert attention from the real issue, which had nothing to do with Ugandans being shipped to Britain for AIDS treatment. The reality was about the moral and legal grounds pertaining to a small number of AIDS patients already in Britain on life-saving treatment being sent back to die. It was about the lives of individuals like the small girl and her mother. The innocent little girl on AIDS treatment in Britain knew nothing about the issue of the huge numbers of AIDS sufferers in a far away country that Dr X was trying to use to dislodge her from her lifeline, presumably as a deterrent to the 1.4 million strong "invasion" force. As a medical practitioner, Dr X knew very well that being infected with HIV did not necessarily mean that one needed ARVs. Even with the over 1 million infected people in Uganda, it was estimated at the time that only about 150,000 were in immediate need of ARV therapy. Even with this smaller number nobody had ever suggested that they be sent to Britain. It would be plain stupid to do so. We were all campaigning for affordable drugs and universal access within Uganda and Africa. Thirdly and sadly, Dr X referred to a British National Formulary publication where he picked out the British AIDS drugs pharmacy prices which were obviously more expensive than the access cost in Uganda but only marginally so. He did not bother to comment on the fact that the Ugandan access cost was still unaffordable and that it was the very reason why the Ugandan AIDS patients in the UK were seeking AIDS asylum. Wisely however, he did not in this edition of his letter refer to the rather embarrassing comments in his earlier letter – like "the free drugs and tests or the best treatment programme in the world."

On 21st July 2000, I promptly wrote to the same official in the British embassy in Kampala to whom Dr X had addressed his letter to protest the treacherous misinformation. I explained that Dr X's talk of free drugs was an unashamed, mean and heartless lie that would outrage patients who suffered excruciatingly, orphans mourning their parents, and numerous families who were nursing their loved ones on their death beds without any medicines. I expressed disappointment that an official who resided in Uganda and had ready access to firsthand information accepted being a conduit for false information aimed at hurting sick people:

> As you are based in Uganda you are in a unique position to know the desperate nature of HIV/AIDS in Uganda and to realise that no salaried Ugandan of whatever position can currently afford it on her/his salary without other extra source. In other words these drugs are as good as not available to even the Uganda "middle class".

I took the opportunity to pay well deserved tribute to the British doctors, lawyers and human rights organisations in UK who worked so hard to save Ugandan lives. I also reiterated the same warning as some British doctors had also issued about the fate that awaited AIDS patients if they were sent to Uganda:

> It is our hope that you realise that life-saving therapy offered to Ugandan patients is an ethical humanitarian right. I hope that no patient gets

sent back on Dr X's wrong information that treatment is either free or affordable in Uganda, because removing such patients to where they cannot access treatment on which their lives depends is as good as sentencing them to a painful death.

I never received a reply. However, it appears that Dr X was neutralised as a credible witness at least for a while as I also copied this letter to a number of other concerned UK lawyers. Within a short time I was to learn the extent of the damage Dr X's letter had caused to the HIV-infected Ugandans on treatment in the UK. Apparently my letters offered a stay of execution to some Ugandans who had exhausted all legal channels and were only awaiting the dates of removal. I learned of one such case through the following letter:

London, 23 November 2000

I am assisting a Ugandan with HIV who faces deportation. His previous solicitors fought a case unsuccessfully in the court to prevent his removal. The case was lost largely on the basis of a letter from Dr X dated 22nd October 1999, on which the Home Office was relying.

I have seen your letter, of 10th April 2000, which comments on Dr X's letter and annexed an up to date price list. I will reargue the case in the light of this evidence.

I should be grateful if you could provide me with an update to your letter of 10th April, including an update price list.

Thank you very much for any help you can give.

The lawyers' woes, and more so those of their Ugandan AIDS clients, seemed to ease, as it became abundantly clear that Dr X's evidence, which the Home Office previously relied upon to throw Ugandans out, was so spurious that any lawyer armed with my letter could punch holes in it. This, however, did not mean that the immigration department had rested the matter. On the contrary, their resolve to find new evidence to get rid of undesirable Ugandan AIDS patients continued. It seems that a search for other sources to provide more robust grounds to base the expulsions of Ugandan AIDS patients on started. I got to know that they had found a new "witness" towards the end of the year 2001. This was heralded as usual by yet a new wave of SOS letters from lawyers, including some who had a year earlier expressed the hope that the nightmare for their clients was over as they showered me with letters of thanks for helping them save the lives of their clients. Now they were back to square one. Some of the lawyers had by this time been corresponding with me for over six years and many others had benefited from my general letters that had been passed on to them. They realised that writing so many letters to them was taking too much of my time and a number of them offered to pay me a fee to compensate for my time. I declined their offer. My job was to tell the truth and save lives, and the truth costs nothing. Saving lives is my mission, my calling, and my profession!

A decade of my work on HIV/AIDS was marked in 2000. During that period I had seen too much suffering and too many deaths of AIDS patients. From 1996 I had seen a small number of my patients who were rich enough to afford AIDS drugs resurrected and survive, but, sadly, I had continued to see huge numbers die excruciatingly because they were too poor to pay the price. I had no doubt that most of the Ugandan AIDS sufferers who had fled to Europe were too poor to afford therapy in Uganda. Incidentally, Dr X had argued that Ugandans who were able to afford the ticket to London could afford AIDS drugs! I excused him in this case, because he did not really know what he was talking about. In 2001 an air ticket to London was equivalent to only three months worth of AIDS drugs and laboratory tests. Yet the drugs had to be taken for life. I knew the fate of all those who returned without sufficient funds to purchase their own drugs. Therefore I had to do all I could to warn of this danger. I just could not accept payment for this very basic humanitarian job. It is the very minimum I would expect of every bona fide doctor anywhere in similar circumstances.

"Who was the cause of this latest round of misery for the Ugandan AIDS patients?" I wondered as new letters appealing for help once more poured in. As usual the new culprit was anonymous. A copy of a letter written by the new source was provided to me by one of the lawyers in the form of an attachment to a letter the Home Office had written to him dismissing his clients' application for extended stay in the UK. The new masked person blackened out his or her name so thoroughly that even the dotted signature line was completely obliterated. Evidently, this person was not proud of the job he or she was doing. This person reminded me of the Biblical Pilate, narrated in Matthew 27, verse 24 that reads:

> Seeing that it did no good but, rather, uproar was arising, Pilate took water and washed his hands before the crowd, saying: "I am innocent of the blood of this man. You yourselves must see to it." Pilate said that as he handed over Jesus for crucifixion as was demanded of him by the crowd. He, however, wished to absolve himself of the heinous deed that he did not agree with.

Likewise this person had gone to extraordinary lengths to erase everything that could even remotely connect him/her to the letter. However, the heading, the Foreign and Commonwealth Office, African Department (Equatorial) was not erased presumably because it was a big enough department to give cover to the individual concerned. Also, it was necessary to indicate to the lawyers that the source was authoritative, and in a position to know what goes on in Africa. The erased details included telephone and fax numbers, email address, and personal address. Unlike Dr X, who wrote a rambling letter, this person selected his/her words very carefully. The letter was brief and crisp:

> *Uganda is in the forefront of African countries in the treatment and prevention of AIDS. The DFID Health and Population adviser based in Kampala has confirmed that all the drugs available under NHS are also obtainable locally, and most are also available at a reduced price through UN funded projects and from bilateral AIDS donor funded programmes. For instance the Mildmay AIDS clinic (outside Kampala) has a large DIFD funded treatment centre. There are presently about 2 million AIDS sufferers in Uganda but the incidence of infection is going down. AIDS can be, and is treated locally in Uganda.*

This person was smart, notwithstanding the fact that there were absolutely no UN, or bilateral AIDS donor projects that provided free ARVs in Uganda at the time. The crucial question as to whether deportees would have access to therapy was evaded completely. There was no explicit mention of free drugs or monitoring tests. Clearly this person did not want to tell lies. Therefore by itself this letter was insufficient evidence to fairly have anyone deported. I could see no reason why this individual was so scared to sign his or her name. The information provided was by and large non-committal. The fact that this worried the author, regardless, suggests that the person did not agree with the job for which the letter was intended, and wanted no direct part of it. However, on a separate sheet of paper that obviously could not be traced to anyone, the Home Office had the real damaging material not unlike that of Dr X, which would provide some basis for deporting the "dodgy" Ugandans. The upset defence lawyer wrote to me and I quote the relevant parts:

> *9 November 2001,*
>
> *... Further, the Home Office here is alleging that "a report compiled by an independent observer of the UNAIDS HIV drug access initiative in Uganda points out that the Uganda government established a non-profit making company called Medical Access (U) Limited in 1998 to deal with the procurement , supply and distribution of HIV/AIDS drugs. The report confirms that drugs for the treatment of Opportunistic Infections and Anti-retroviral Therapy (ARV) are supplied to Medical Access (U) Limited at discount prices ...*

Can an average Ugandan now access antiretroviral therapy in Uganda? The short answer was a big NO! With regard to the glorified "UNAIDS HIV drug access initiative, the non-profit company and the Medical Access (U) limited," the amazing details are covered in special sections below. In my view programmes should have been entitled "AIDS drugs Access circus, Accelerated deception, and Donation in a lady's handbag", as some of the details are very upsetting. As described later, this was part of the reason why I had to try and do something about the situation regardless of the consequences.

Up until 2002 no major donor had ever made any meaningful antiretroviral drugs donation to Uganda or any other African country, despite the sham claims above. While it is true that the British Development Fund for International Development (DFID) helped in setting up Mildmay, when it came to antiretroviral drugs their contribution was about nil, just like all other rich Western countries. Interestingly, with one cheek, Uganda was being described colourfully as "a world leader in AIDS treatment delivered by leading world experts" so as to get rid of Ugandan AIDS patients from Europe, while with another it was said gloomily that "AIDS drugs are too complicated to be used in Africa, as they lack even the very basic expertise and infrastructure" so as explain away the millions of preventable deaths of Africans. Meanwhile Africa was being denied even the very basic opportunities for research on AIDS drugs through which some patients could have accessed the life-saving therapy on the pretext that "AIDS research in Africa was impossible.

Meanwhile, AIDS deaths in Africa had by 2001 hit a new record. All these deaths happened when life-saving drugs had long been discovered, but were being denied to the dying poor in Uganda and Africa at large. That on top of this the UK immigration department's determination to remove desperate AIDS patients on the bogus pretext that life-saving treatment would be easily and freely available to them in Uganda was to say the least disheartening. However, I do not believe that Ugandans were a specific target group. It could have happened to any group of Africans AIDS patients.

Rich Orphan, Poor Orphan

To treat or not to treat is the question

The poor HIV infected children deported from UK would have joined the pool of the most pathetic of all patients who I encountered. Among the heartrending cases were children that endured the double jeopardy of being both helpless orphans and also sufferers of AIDS. One such orphan was a young boy aged 7, whom I will name Baguma in order to protect his identity. AIDS had wiped out many of his relatives, leaving no one in his extended family capable of taking care of him. However, with a rare stroke of luck, an amazingly resourceful woman I call Jovanis found him in distress and undertook to foster him. Jovanis first introduced Baguma to me when he was so seriously sick that it was doubtful whether he would survive the next few weeks. Indeed many prospective foster parents would have distanced themselves from such a child, because he would be too much trouble to nurse, as he would need full time attention, yet in the end all efforts would prove futile. But to this woman this was more of a reason to take him in. I was to learn later that in fact Baguma was just one of the ten other homeless orphans and destitute children that Jovanis had under her care. She was able to feed, clothe, and pay for their schooling without a paying job or any sort of regular income except for a small subsistence farm in *Bunyaruguru,* in a rural southern Uganda village bordering Queen Elizabeth National Park. In the small farm, she grew seasonal crops including bananas, millet, beans and potatoes mainly for home consumption leaving a small surplus to sell in the local market to provide for her and the children. However, Jovanis frequently lost all her crops. The menace came from animals, especially elephants and baboons that frequently escaped from the nearby game reserve and ruined her gardens, leaving her to scavenge for food. Yet this did not stop her from taking on more children and also helping out with some other poor AIDS patients in her village. I once asked her why she was doing all this even at the cost of self-denial.

"God blessed me with a gift, of helping others in distress," Jovanis a devout Catholic replied, "and besides I cannot stand a suffering child. It just breaks my heart."

Oh! How Africa desperately needed such hundreds of thousands of the blessed ones!

Baguma was infected with HIV at birth and no one knew it until he came down with an extensive skin rash characterised by small papules with depression that looked like a belly button in the middle known to doctors as *Molluscum contageosum.* This was caused by a skin virus infection brought about by his lowered immune system. However, when I first saw him he had progressed to full-blown AIDS, and in most urgent need of the life saving antiretroviral therapy (ART) for his very survival. The dilemma, as it were, was the highly astronomical cost of the drugs that Baguma desperately needed to stay alive. It was far over and above Jovanis's means - actually she had almost no means. The treatment cost at the time was unaffordable to the vast majority of even most well-to-do Ugandans. Therefore, in the case of

Jovanis it was just not an option. It would have been madness for her to even contemplate starting Baguma on AIDS drugs, because by the mid-1990s the cost of only two weeks AIDS drugs was equivalent to Jovanis's entire income for one year from her peasant farm. Yet the treatment was needed to save his life. To add to that, it looked like he had almost reached a point of no return, as he was clearly in the advanced stage of AIDS, very weak, emaciated and suffering from multiple life-threatening opportunistic infections. Yet incredibly and against all odds Jovanis just went ahead and found the money to get him started on the prohibitively expensive AIDS drugs. Almost everyone advised her against this option considering the huge cost, but she just would not listen. Having found money for the drugs at least in the short term it was virtually impossible to deny him the treatment, though it looked more like a stay of execution than sustainable therapy. Baguma responded wonderfully well to treatment, and was resurrected from the abyss. His strength slowly returned, as did the smile to his face. He began to put on some flesh on his skinny bones, and within a few months, the miracle was complete! He was well enough to return to school as Jovanis dashed in all directions looking for more money to maintain him on the therapy.

She told me of her remarkable story of self-determination, which included camping outside the president's office insisting on seeing the Presidential Welfare Officer for help. On several occasions the indomitable woman made it to the President himself to request him for assistance. President Museveni, renowned for compassion towards AIDS victims, ordered the welfare officer to give her every possible assistance. However, there were too many destitute and desperate people all being supported on the president's relatively small welfare budget and so there was not enough to go round. Jovanis had to look elsewhere for the necessary supplement.

Unfortunately but not surprisingly, even Jovanis's zeal and determination was not enough to ensure uninterrupted supplies of antiretroviral drugs yet it was absolutely crucial for successful AIDS treatment. As a result the boy often missed doses simply because she would sometimes fail to find the money in time. Inevitably the dreaded antiretroviral treatment catastrophe happened. Baguma developed resistance to the AIDS drugs. Yet these were the simplest, most user-friendly, and the cheapest available. Now that they were no longer working for him, the only alternative was to change to the second line drugs. This change, in terms of cost and complexity, was like jumping from the frying pan right into the fire. First of all, the cost of the second line drugs was more than double the cost of the first, making it as many times more difficult to get the money to pay for them. On top of that, the new drugs necessitated increased numbers of pills (the pill burden) that Baguma had to take daily. The new therapy included a recent class of drugs known as protease inhibitors (PI), which was associated with more unpleasant side effects so making tolerability much more difficult for him. However, the main constraint by far remained the exorbitant cost of the drugs. At the time, it seemed to me that the boy's fate was sealed, as Jovanis was clearly caught between a rock and a hard place. I recall having a lengthy painful discussion with her that left me feeling ruffled. It was apparent from our discussions that the problems facing Jovanis were insurmountable. This spelt only doom for the hapless boy. I, therefore, enlisted the help of one of our counsellors to discuss the situation with both her and Baguma, and to prepare both of them for the inevitable, or as it was often coded, encourage them to "live positively."

Thanks to the power of antiretroviral drugs that had restored his immune system, Baguma was not in immediate danger. I advised Jovanis to avoid re-starting him on therapy as she was bound to do if she managed to get some little money. I told her that treatment was useless unless she was sure that it would be sustained. Fortunately Baguma remained well for a year but then inevitably symptoms started creeping back as AIDS resurged. Once more he weakened and the death clock countdown once more started ticking. It was now just a matter of time - a rather short time!

To my amazement, the unbelievable Jovanis once again turned up demanding treatment for the ailing boy. "I have found the money for the drugs," she said as she stretched out her hands holding a neat bundle of one thousand shillings notes. "Doctor you need to be fast.

Baguma is now very sick, and I am afraid he won't have long to live unless you save him." Jovanis had raised only enough money for about five months of treatment. I could now visualise the same futile scenario playing all over once again. I had to be careful what I said to her, because she seemed least prepared to take 'no' as an answer. Yet it was the right one in the dire circumstances.

"You have done very well to come up with five months' treatment," I tentatively started to explain, trying to use only the right words, "but five months is a very short time in the treatment of a chronic illness."

"Well, that's five months head start to look for the follow-on money," she interjected. "If Baguma is not put on therapy now he will not be alive in five months, too late for you to know if I would get more money or not," she added, leaving me no alternative that I could live with but to re-start him on therapy.

Admittedly, in so doing I had no hesitation because her reasoning was sensible and deep inside me I was cheering for the boy's survival. I must admit that a loving woman struggling to save an innocent young gift of life from a marauding scourge touched me. By that time I was also looking at Jovanis with a heightened sense of awe for her remarkable resilience. Naturally curiosity got the better of me and I wanted to know a bit more about her background, because she was an extraordinary being. However, I found that she was not the type who wanted to talk much about herself or dwell too much on past events. However, I was able to gather that she was not always so insolvent.

The sixty-six year old woman was born into a well-to-do family, of a Saza (county) chief in the then Kingdom of Ankole, before the kingdom was abolished by President Obote in 1966. Since then her fortunes took amazing turns and twists that saw this remarkable woman in different roles. However, due to past political turmoil in Uganda the trend was from riches to rags. At the end of it all, she emerged ever so smart in a simple sort of way, polite to a fault, yet engaging and hassle-free. I could see that she must have been a great beauty in her youth, a fact confirmed by her contemporaries. No wonder at one time she worked for and fitted well in a beauty shop, called Grayson and Company that sold cosmetics and other women's make-up in the 1960s. Men chased after her in her youth, but I was told that Jovanis had a way of putting unwelcome suitors off, counselling them without generating offence and still retained some of them as friends despite the pain of being snubbed. By the early 1960s she had also rediscovered her talents as a natural leader and campaigner in the wake of her increasing interest in politics.

As an intelligent, sociable and beautiful woman that stood out among others, she caught the eye of one of the Ugandan kings and ended up in the palace as a companion. She was to become a close confidante of the king, and in turn helped him politically. Jovanis was so appreciated, that his majesty would occasionally put on some disguise just for the pleasure of chauffeuring her himself. She was well recognised as part of the royal entourage until 1966, when all the Ugandan tribal kingdoms were abolished. What followed was a very difficult time for Jovanis while she watched helplessly as the king was dethroned, and her world fell apart. However, she was good at picking up the pieces and married a senior army officer, but the marriage did not work out and they separated in 1974. Jovanis then seemed to disappear, but resurfaced as an active member and campaigner for Museveni's Uganda Patriotic Movement (UPM) party, in the 1980 elections which were lost. Jovanis then kept a low profile to avoid harassment by the victorious Uganda Peoples Congress (UPC) as Museveni launched the bush war from 1981 to 1986, to oust Obote who was accused of rigging the election. Jovanis was said to have been of some unspecified clandestine assistance to the rebel army. From what I gather about Jovanis and what I saw of her, she was definitely the kind of person you would want on your side when fighting a tough war.

Jovanis saw first hand all the turmoil Uganda went through, including Amin's brutal regime, the wars that created chaos in the country, and the AIDS scourge, some of which adversely affected her own family. Her calm manners and self-evident resilience could be her way of masking some personal painful experiences and the lessons learned. She never had children of her own, but whatever it was that she lost as a mother she more than made up for as a foster parent. The soft-spoken woman successfully fundraised for her orphaned foster children's needs. In over ten years that I have known Jovanis, I never saw her upset, rattled or in any way appear overwhelmed by the obviously heavy burden of the many children she shouldered. She just acted as if taking care of children was just the natural thing to do. However, I found her an incredibly determined fighter for her children. She was just not a quitter.

This time, Jovanis miraculously managed to get the huge amount of money to pay for the expensive drugs on a more regular basis. The records confirmed that she was always collecting drugs on schedule. However, Baguma's treatment monitoring tests did not look good. Something was not quite right. I asked Jovanis to find out what the problem could be. It eventually turned out that Baguma was not actually taking the drugs regularly because they made him sick. He would collect the tablets but always made a quick movement like he was throwing them into the mouth, only to briskly swing his hand round and put the distasteful tablets smartly in his pocket. He would then throw them away later when no one was looking. When Jovanis started watching him more carefully while he took the drugs he would often throw up. I tried changing his therapy in an attempt to get some combination that could be better tolerated but to no avail as the choice was limited.

I arranged for extra counselling for him, but he always pleaded that he would very much like to take the drugs but he could not help being made sick by them. Anyway, he pursued on under his foster mother's patient supervision and in time he seemed to get used to the drugs. Then he stabilised and became well enough to continue with schooling. A year later, he requested to go to a boarding school, but I initially advised her not to let him go unless she was absolutely sure that his therapy would be supervised. In fact, Jovanis shared my concerns and was clearly not happy to have him out of her sight. She also had another good reason for not wishing him to go to the boarding school. She feared he would be stigmatised by other children and possibly teachers as well, if they found out that he had AIDS. Yet at least some of the teachers had to know since they had to administer the drugs. But Baguma himself insisted that he very much wanted to go to a boarding school just like other kids of his age and kept begging her to let him go. In addition, he had developed an interest in sports and liked to play football and take part in outdoor activities. Jovanis visited the school and discussed these difficult issues with the teachers. They were sympathetic and reassured her that the school would supervise his treatment. I would have expected nothing less as many Ugandan teachers were themselves living with HIV/AIDS. Like all other Ugandans, almost all would have had family members or relatives of their own infected or affected by HIV.

Baguma got to like the boarding school very much and coped well, although his academic performance was initially below average. His school reports talked of "a very well behaved child who liked sports though he was frequently disturbed by recurrent infections." I was pleased to see him grow into a lovely handsome boy. Then some lengthy interval passed without him coming back to the clinic. The next time I saw him I could not believe my eyes! Baguma was so sick that he needed urgent hospitalisation. He had just returned from a school trip to neighbouring Kenya. While there, he came down with a serious chest infection. Fortunately he responded well to antibiotic treatment, but when I checked his blood I found that he had developed resistance even to the second line HIV drugs. This was very bad news.

The only alternative therapy left for poor Baguma was the so-called Salvage Therapy, which means that no standard ART treatment regimen would be effective. At this stage the only thing that can be done is try everything available in the hope that somehow it may be of some help. This therefore meant that Baguma had to take more pills and correspondingly suffer more side-effects than ever before. On Jovanis's side, this meant that her problems had further multiplied. Firstly, the new treatment regimen was much more expensive. Then she was faced with the titanic battle of getting Baguma to take the "abominable" pills. It was indeed a painful experience, which often ended in anguish for both her and Baguma, as he had great difficulty keeping the drugs down. The ever patient woman cajoled and encouraged him to keep on trying, fully aware that the alternative was death.

The way antiretroviral drugs were used by Baguma would shock any Western doctor blessed with easy access to AIDS drugs, and patients who had no problems affording them. I knew a number of Western professionals who advocated denial of drugs to Africa precisely because they feared that what befell Baguma would happen on such a massive scale that it would make all AIDS drugs useless due to widespread HIV resistance. The West feared that the resistant virus would shift from Africa to their own doorsteps – rekindling the disease that had by and large been efficiently controlled in their part of the world, and create a problem for the people there. Some voices strongly advocated not using the drugs at all on patients in Africa unless there was a guarantee that they would first ensure uninterrupted drugs supplies for life and guarantee adherence, and demonstrate clear understanding of the complicated regimen. In mid-1990s, whenever I reported that we had a substantial number of patients on the new ART drugs in Uganda, I was always asked: "How do you make sure that your patients can afford and sustain treatment? How much money do they have to have before you can start them on treatment?" The questions were always asked with a thinly disguised tone of disapproval. I can imagine what may have been said behind my back. However, no answer seemed to satisfy the sceptics. As far as some of our privileged colleagues from the West were concerned, their view was that no patient should be started on ARVs unless capacity to sustain treatment indefinitely was clearly demonstrated and documented. For all but a very tiny minority of our patients, this was virtually impossible.

Such disciples would have recommended that the likes of Jovanis should have been told in no uncertain terms that putting Baguma on therapy was a hopeless battle, not worth trying. Her sentiments would have been ignored completely. They would argue that she would be too busy nursing him through the agonies of recurrent infections to think too much about antiretroviral therapy. After all, without ART he would have died within a couple of months or may be a year at the most. Jovanis would have presumably moaned for a few weeks and, like millions of others, come to terms with her tragic loss, as she nursed the next child in the pipeline of death. As I tried to find some more affordable drugs, I met many people, especially those associated with the donor community and pharmaceutical business, who would just shake their heads, as if to say "in such dire circumstances where nothing could be done, "living positively" while waiting for the inevitable was all that was feasible for the poor patients." In their view ART was just not an option. In the meantime, alternative but useless therapies were extensively recommended for HIV treatment in poor countries. Books and pamphlets were widely published, allegedly written by experts on AIDS treatment in poor countries. What was actually missing in such publications was AIDS treatment itself. Instead there were apologies, factual omissions and coded language. For instance, overtly poor countries ceased to be referred to as such. They were instead renamed "resource constrained" or the other politically correct name of "developing countries," even though AIDS had reversed almost all development that had been achieved over the previous twenty years. The basically useless "supportive" drugs recommended for the poor were described in positive terms despite being totally ineffective as far as AIDS was concerned. Even use of 'traditional medicines' was encouraged though there was no such thing as traditional medicine against AIDS. The disease was as new to the traditional medicine as it was to Western medicine. Many donors turned a blind eye as Africans in their desperation consumed tons of soil, vitamins, ineffective herbs and other strange concoctions.

Without ARVs, Baguma would have probably died by 1997, but over eight years later in 2006, he remains fairly well and attends a boarding secondary school. Almost all other children of his age with AIDS in Uganda were denied the gift of life. On the other hand, Baguma has lived a reasonably tolerable life for the last eight years though admittedly he has suffered some bad side effects due to the drugs, and because he fell into drug misuse, almost unavoidable in such a dire state of poverty. If he had been rich, early drugs resistance would have been avoided. Poverty just makes adherence impossible unless the drugs are affordable, or free.

The exorbitant cost of life-saving drugs made them inaccessible to the poor, and forced people like Baguma to resort to desperate measures. Jovanis had a right to fight for her child's life. And she did it amazingly well by fighting tooth and nail but she was always destined to fail in the end. True, the pharmaceutical companies did not go out of their way to hurt poor Baguma personally. As individuals the big Pharma workers feel exactly the same as anyone else, and indeed most of those I have met are as compassionate as any other human being. Some actually extended some help, albeit small. However, at corporate level, the system of competition, and anonymity behind big companies, as well as other strategic interests, drives them to prioritise returns, while issues related to human suffering at least as far as AIDS and diseases of the poor were concerned, are left in the background.

Failure to ensure uninterrupted access to ART is perhaps the single most important threat to the successful use of ARVs in Africa. It is likely to lead to widespread development of AIDS drugs resistance that may spiral out of control. As the pharmaceutical industry and WTO have an important role in the determination and enforcement of international trade laws like TRIPS or patents laws, they therefore bear primary responsibility to find a way forward. This will minimise the chances of widespread drugs resistance and a fate similar to what happened to Baguma.

So what remained of hapless Baguma's fate now that he had multi-drug resistance and the only available drugs were too expensive, besides being almost impossible for him to take? From December 2003, there was some good and bad news for him. The good news was that he became one of the first beneficiaries, and deservedly so, of the first free drugs access programme in Uganda. Nowadays, Jovanis does not have to suffer the anguish of begging, and scavenging for Baguma's drugs anymore. Further good news is that science has made available some newer drugs that have helped reduce the pill burden and that in turn helps Baguma as far as compliance is concerned. On a comforting note, especially for Jovanis, even with his resistant virus, Baguma's disease is not progressing, and clinically he remains stable. Unless one has prior knowledge about Baguma's HIV status, one is unable to tell the ordeal he has gone through even when he is at school. His grades have improved and he has recently been promoted in class. However, the bad news is that he has to await development of newer drugs to ensure he gets ones that will work really well for him again.

Talking about the need for new drugs provides a good propaganda opportunity for the pharmaceutical companies. "See, you need new drugs," they respond. "If you do not allow us to recoup our cost of developing life saving drugs, then this is what you get. There will just be no new drugs for you. This way you just kill innovation." I have heard this excuse countless times. Many other people do not relate it to the wider implications. It has become the main rallying threat used to justify profiteering at any cost, even if millions of lives are sacrificed. Obviously no sensible person wants to kill the goose that lays the golden pills. However, the current trade policies that do not balance profits and critical life and death situations are not essentially in the long-term interests of either patients or the pharmaceutical industry.

Bad as Baguma's situation was, he had a woman of steel to fend for him. His situation, though harrowing, could be described as heavenly in comparison to a heartbreak child I call Joy, whose agonising ordeal still haunts me. Joy was a pleasant highly intelligent girl who was always top of her class. She got HIV from her mother and by the age of four both her parents had died of AIDS, leaving her a double orphan. She was left under the care of her aunt, who was married to a fairly prosperous businessman. The caring couple had five other children of their own, but were endowed with two cars, a good house and all the basic amenities of life. By Ugandan standards they were a very rich couple. Joy used to be brought to my clinic in a shiny new car, suffering from one Opportunistic Infection after another despite being on Septrin prophylaxis. One day, taking advantage of the rare privacy with me provided by her aunt going out briefly, Joy asked me to explain to her why she was always falling sick.

I replied that I needed to discuss this issue with her auntie first and together we would then discuss it with her. When I put this to the aunt, she was strongly against disclosure of the grim diagnosis. I reasoned the child needed to know the reason why, unlike other children, she was always taking many bitter pills and still not getting well. At least we needed to give an explanation that made sense to her. I pointed out that the child was bright enough to understand and would even handle her situation better if she knew the diagnosis. The aunt, however ,remained insistent that she did not approve of disclosure to her niece. "It would devastate her," she pleaded.

When Joy, who had been waiting outside the room while I discussed her fate with her aunt, returned, she evidently expected an explanation – a good one. I told her that her body was weak and not able to fight the diseases like other kids at school. She asked why her body was weak. I replied that she was born with it. Then she asked whether there was a medicine to make her better. "Yes," I replied.

"But it keeps coming back," she insisted.

"It is because the medicines I give you do not work on your body weakness which makes you catch so many infections. It only deals with each infection as it comes." I explained trying to be as truthful as possible.

I thought I could see glitter in her eyes as she thought about the delicate problem. "Doctor, why don't you give me the medicine for the body weakness instead?" she pleaded. Her aunt and I just eyed each other in uneasy silence!

"Such a medicine does not exist," her aunt finally lied to her.

"Then I will keep falling sick," she said. Her aunt kept quiet, as I shifted uneasily in my chair. "Is it true doctor?" she asked me. I had really hoped that I would not be put on the spot! I hate lying to my patients. And I couldn't. Instead I chose to answer another question, which I was not asked. "You need to keep taking the medicines whenever the illness comes," I said to her, really feeling very bad that this child was not being told the whole story. "Thank you doctor," she said. "I will be a good girl and take my medicines." She finally kindly let me off the hook. "I promise," she added.

The medicines that were being prescribed for Joy at the very best only afforded her temporary relief. In between she was always in pain. The pain was not inevitable. Neither were the horrific opportunistic infections she repeatedly suffered from. Her misery could have been stopped with antiretroviral drugs. Instead she was being treated with drugs that did not solve the real problem of her body's weakness. Unlike what her aunt told her, drugs did indeed exist, but as long as they were not accessible they were as good as non-existent. So once again, in that context her aunt was perhaps right.

I tried all my best to persuade the aunt to dig deep into her pockets and put Joy on ART, but made no headway. I tried to get the aunt to organise a fundraising drive, but after a while she came back to report that it had failed. She was adamant that the therapy was just too expensive. She had her own children at school, and the family was used to a standard of living that would have been greatly affected if she offered to pay the cost of Joy's drugs.

Joy paid the cost with her life.

The terminal stage of her illness was most distressing to all of us who helplessly watched her in agony. Until she lapsed into coma she could not let go of her bottle of Septrin, keeping her solemn promise to be a good girl. The end came almost as a God sent relief, as she succumbed to AIDS just like the hundreds of thousands of other unfortunate children in Africa.

The contrast between the case of Joy, the rich orphan, and that of Baguma, the poor one, under the care of Jovanis the almost penniless woman, is most paradoxical. Most likely under Jovanis, Joy too would still be alive but she would almost certainly have developed drugs resistance. The aunt certainly loved her niece but considered the necessary sacrifice too disruptive to her own family. Jovanis, on the other hand, would have scavenged around and started her on therapy regardless. When Joy died the aunt was devastated - genuinely. I had a bit of sympathy for her and some degree of understanding based on my personal experience. With so many children in similar circumstances under my care - at one time an entire children's ward - it was an almost daily painful experience to see them die, knowing pretty well that they could have lived if only they had access to drugs.

However, I kept thinking that Joy's aunt could have survived the sacrifice of getting her niece treated. This was until I chanced to meet her several months later. I must confess that I had felt an inner anger for this otherwise very kind and pleasant woman because I considered her rather heartless. When I chanced to meet her, I couldn't help inquiring how she was handling the loss, by way of trying to get an explanation as to why she was seemingly so callous by declining to make the life saving ART available to poor Joy. She just broke into tears. Obviously she too was living the nightmare of Joy's demise. In her case a double tragedy, because of lingering remorse.

"We are overwhelmed with so many AIDS patients in our family," she said sobbing. "We do not even know where to start with ART, because we would have to sacrifice everything we have." She now looked me straight in the eye and added, "And even if we sold all our possessions, we still would not manage to treat even half of those who need the life-saving drugs in our family"

Well, she was not alone! All of us in "resource constrained" countries were in the same boat. I felt ashamed that I had insensitively judged her harshly. I understood. I forgave her. However, I found my mind wondering back to the painful period, and inevitably to Joy's well-attended church funeral service. I just had to be there to say a final farewell to her as I braced myself to meet many others in similar situation. Though one of many, this special child made me bleed inside. I was asked to say a few words to the mourners, but I was short of words. I did say something lamenting the tragic death of such a brilliant little girl, but what I remember most vividly is a throat filling surging anger, shame and frustration that I felt, seeing so many people coming to attend the funeral of one little girl, instead of all of us pulling together in the first place to prevent her death. Although numerous others were out there crying aloud for the same, it just looked like this one was really a special child that needed to be saved.

I just could not help thinking that something needed to be done about the cost of drugs. It was the main cause of misery and deaths for the likes of Baguma who could access the drugs but not sustain them for life, and those like Joy who could not access them and died excruciatingly. Unless the affordable pricing of drugs for life-threatening diseases became an international standard, a huge number of Joys would inevitably continue to die, while a huge number of Baguma's would develop widespread AIDS drugs resistance. We know very well how to fight and minimise drugs resistance. It is by strict adherence. Adherence, however, is impossible without easy access to drugs. A Catch-22 situation!

Pharmaceutical companies should help poor countries avert the hovering threat of the emergence of resistance to their own AIDS drugs. By way of justification, some apologists have pointed out that there is widespread resistance to drugs for tropical diseases like malaria despite the cost of drugs being relatively cheap. "Therefore it is not the cost that is the problem," some conclude. This kind of reasoning, however, is flawed. We are forewarned from experience and more advanced knowledge that drug misuse, which caused widespread resistance like that to anti-malaria drugs, could be minimised. Therefore, we do not have to fall in the same pit twice if we take good care. All that is needed is to institute robust measures to fight the misuse of AIDS drugs because they are even more delicate than malaria drugs. We must be on the watch for channels that tend to fast-track resistance. However, we need the co-operation of the big Pharma because, contrary to what is said, the main culprit for misuse of drugs remains their excessive cost.

Nevertheless, a vigorous programme to ensure adherence must be instituted, especially as donor-funded drugs are introduced, because this is quite critical. It must include public information, education and communication. People with a life-threatening disease like AIDS cannot be stopped from trying to access life-saving therapy. As long as the drugs remain too expensive, or are not guaranteed to be accessible all the time, they will be misused because they cannot be sustained in their proper use. One could weirdly argue that those like Joy who fail to access the delicate AIDS drugs do not contribute to resistance since they just die off, and to some extent this is correct but very disturbing. This cannot justify denial of life-saving drugs to millions of desperate poor people, because it is not only unethical but also a gross violation of basic human rights.

It is genocide by denial.

Survival is for the Rich

Throughout the 1990s I faced a complex dilemma involving the huge numbers of poor and desperately ill AIDS patients, who swarmed my clinic and the JCRC, yet almost always left empty-handed simply because they were too poor to afford the ransom demanded by the makers of the life-saving drugs. The predicament was that no donor would fund antiretroviral therapy or even subsidise it as this was then a no-go funding area described often as "a bottomless pit." The only ARV drugs available in the country were those that I had managed to import using very limited funds I raised from a small section of my patients who had the means to purchase their own drugs on cost-recovery basis.

I am still haunted by a distressing meeting with one relative I call Paulo Barya, a peasant from my home southern district of Rukungiri. I vividly recall the encounter as if it was just yesterday as Paulo staggered into my office that extraordinary Monday afternoon in June 1998. Apparently Paulo had heard about the new AIDS drugs, and personally witnessed a miracle whereby a village trader at death's door was raised from the dead by the wonder drugs. Paulo heard it whispered that the doctor who had pulled off this miracle was his own cousin – myself. Sniffing a lifeline, Paulo quickly marshalled transport money by selling some foodstuffs he could hardly afford to do without, and made a beeline for Kampala City to look for me. After a gruelling six-hour bus journey, an emaciated, hungry and very tired Paulo staggered into my office unannounced, at about 2.30 in the afternoon. He collapsed his bony frame into a chair sighing with both relief and exhaustion. Speaking wearily, while taking deep breaths in between short phrases, he initially beat about the bush, as is the cultural etiquette, narrating some uncoordinated news of the state of health of various relatives in the village, even though none was so sick as himself, before addressing the main reason of his visit. "As you can see, I don't have long to live unless you help me out," Paulo finally stuttered. "I gather you have stumbled upon a cure - and I have come for it."

Paulo was absolutely spot on as far as his self-diagnosis was concerned. An old shingles scar on the right side of his face that blinded his right eye, his pale scanty hair, extensive skin rash with scratch marks all over, white coated tongue and gross emaciation confirmed that indeed Paulo was in advanced stages of AIDS. Patients in such a state normally have a few months to a year to live at the very best. That is unless they can immediately access antiretroviral therapy. I painstakingly explained that I did not personally have the life saving drugs that he needed. It was, of course, useless discussing the huge cost involved with him, considering that he did not even have money for his meals, his transport money back home notwithstanding. As he was aware that the drugs that would lift his death sentence were indeed stocked in our pharmacy, I had to give him a really good reason why they were not accessible to him although he so desperately needed them. In as simple terms as possible, I conscientiously explained that the cost of the drugs was unaffordable.

"Why do they make them so expensive when they are supposed to save lives?" asked Paulo, who obviously was unaware of the complexities of pharmaceutical trade. I explained that the pharmaceutical companies determined the prices. Still Paulo found this explanation unsatisfactory, and I reluctantly felt obliged to give him the usual pharmaceutical rhetoric. I apologised that I had no sufficient personal resources to buy him drugs. But Paulo was either not listening or did not care for my explanations. Perhaps his mind was focussed on his critical fight for survival. His dilemma was surely understandable. Here he was so close to the life-saving ART, yet so far away, like a starving cow in a bare paddock with lush green grass on the other side of the fence. This is a heart wrenching experience for any physician to face: A dying patient denied urgently needed life-saving therapy perfectly legally under international law!

This whole thing must have sounded just like mumbo-jumbo to him. Old desperate Paulo at the end of his tether was not making it easy for me.

"Please excuse me brother, I am not well enough to listen to so many of your stories," he pleaded despairingly. "All I need is the drug to save my life. It is my last hope." He paused briefly to take a laboured breath, and then added, "And after I have regained my usual well known sense of humour, I promise I can crack much better jokes."

Unfortunately for poor Paulo, there was nothing funny. His village was about to lose a great storyteller and humorist. The reality was that as a poor man with AIDS he had no alternative but to prepare to endure more pain and suffering. He would eventually turn into a statistic which would, if he were lucky, be picked up by UNAIDS and posted on the world's skyrocketing death toll. All that was accessible to the likes of Paulo was counselling - for all that it was worth, and Septrin. Counselling was an easy option, and generally not taken seriously as a discipline of healthcare. Anyone could become a counsellor. This in itself was not necessarily out of order, because all they had to do in absence of ART was to help patients die without crying out too loudly. The donors had invested a lot in counselling as the only intervention for the poor AIDS patients in Africa. In standardised counselling sessions, Paulo would be advised to "live positively." The counsellor would exalt the virtues of upholding a positive attitude and remaining committed to the same principle even if the going got tough, as it inevitably would, on his painful march to the AIDS slaughterhouse. For enlightened Paulo, it would surely be hard to live positively when he knew very well that he could do better than that if only he could get his hands on the magic drugs. It was not far away. It was right here in Uganda, at the JCRC, under the custody of a relative. Rich people had unlimited access to it. They did not have to just "live positively." Instead they lived normally or as close to normalcy as possible. The poor had to be good boys and girls, living positively waiting for a peaceful exit - and not crying out loud.

It was ironic that the resource-constrained countries with a huge AIDS burden had no AIDS drugs, while the rich Western countries with a small number of patients had the lion's share. The ludicrous nature of the excuses for this situation could have been easily dismissed as just the selfish mutterings of pharmaceutical rhetoric, but were often lent credence by many respectable and highly qualified people who ought to have known better and perhaps did. These were keynote speakers at international AIDS conferences, the state-of-the-art lecturers at seminars, and the conveners of forums and major decision-making bodies. They talked of treating poor people with ART as if it was rocket science, described conditions in developing countries as if it was a different planet, and portrayed the essential conditions for safe and effective use of ARVs as virtually unattainable in poor countries. Many unwittingly became apologists and spokesmen for the status quo and inadvertently participated in denial or delayed rescue for at least some of the suffering patients. The hyped-up sophistication associated with antiretroviral therapy was deliberately grossly exaggerated.

Notwithstanding the widespread poverty in most African rural areas, the situation was made to demonstrate a much more chaotic situation than the reality. The infrastructure constraint was projected as just insurmountable. The high level of adherence necessary for optimum ART outcome as well as minimisation of the emergency of HIV resistance was said to be just unachievable in Africa. In some diversionary moves, "experts" recommended that considering the dire conditions in Africa, mere provision of clean water was more of an urgent priority, arguing that it would save many more AIDS patients' lives than would ARVs. Some gullible people took this mean joke literally. Some went as far as diverting emergency life-saving AIDS drugs money to provide drinking water to AIDS patients instead. Some are still doing so today! If the provision of water was so critically important (as indeed it is in all countries), one would have expected serious investment in the construction of protected wells and the provision of piped water to the dry area and the congested slum. However, no such programmes were undertaken. Instead, mainly easy and token options, were offered such as the provision of clay pots to "keep water cool". These were the kind of interventions Africans could do for themselves while donors concentrated on more urgent interventions like providing the life-saving drugs which was beyond Africa's means.

If the soon-to-die Paulo had the misfortune to learn what was really going on, and the real reasons why he was being denied the vital drugs, he would have thought that the world had gone crazy. All he had to say in anger and disappointment by way of farewell to me, as he prepared to return to the village to await the unbearable was: "I know that you have the drugs in this institution that could save my life." Paulo admonished me, "Are you so pitiless as to send me back home empty-handed to die?" Tough! Paulo was smart enough to know that without ART, his life was precariously poised, but he could not see that I was not his executioner. "I put my death on your shoulders" Paulo pushed in the stab, leaving me morose and introspective. The sting still lingers on long after Paulo's death.

My predicament, for which I forgave Paulo for not appreciating, was that, by the end of that very day I would have seen between ten and thirty others in desperate need of the same drugs just like him, and by the end of the week they would run into hundreds. Across Uganda there were over a million and a half living with HIV/AIDS, and perhaps over 200,000 in immediate need of the life-saving drugs. He did not realise that by the end of the year, millions would have died of AIDS in Africa. But on a more personal note the twenty or so close poor relatives, including Paulo, who had approached me in need of ART within that week alone, would have cost me about $200,000 per year, which would have taken me forty-four years to earn on my salary. Paulo was not aware that if I needed the medicines myself, I like him, could not afford it. At national level, if Uganda were to provide free ART for all the 200,000 people it would have cost over 2 billion dollars per year. Although Uganda was experiencing rapid economic recovery, it was then managing to export goods worth just over $400 million per annum. As for the entire Sub-Saharan Africa, close to twenty million were living with HIV and about 15% of them were in immediate need of ART. It does not take a genius to work out that the drugs' cost would have been prohibitively huge. The message, which the invested interests propagated, using these monstrous statistics as an apology for this quagmire, was that problems associated with AIDS treatment in Africa were just insoluble and therefore nobody's fault. I often saw many of my fellow colleagues, thoroughly mesmerised and bewildered by these mind-boggling figures. Some just threw up their arms in total resignation, saying, "Well, that's it!" At every AIDS seminar or conference, specially selected keynote speakers would rattle these staggering figures out. Glossy leaflets would be liberally distributed to make absolutely sure that the message conveyed by the dreadful data was driven home and remain ringing in the ears loud and clear.

If you dared present these figurers to a dying man like Paulo, he probably would have thought you were from Mars. Knowing Paulo's sharp mind and wit, I bet he would have retorted, "I am one dying human being in need of help and not a statistic." This indeed would have been my honest position too, if I were in his shoes. I have never been impressed by such gruesome figures. To me, they represented the horror and scope of the tragedy, and an imperative for an immediate massive international response. Sadly humans react to emergencies fast if they are vividly dramatic, like the collapse of a building or an earthquake. On December, 26,2004, a devastating earthquake with the epicentre in the Indian Ocean near Indonesia triggered a devastating tsunami that hit the coastal areas of southern Asia that also spread as far away as the East African coast. Within forty-eight hours close to 60,000 people were confirmed dead and the numbers were still rising to eventually run into hundreds of thousands. The report talked of the biggest emergency rescue mission in history. All the rich nations quickly responded with unprecedented pledges, which ran into billions of dollars in immediate relief. Resources were swiftly mobilised and the USA dispatched two battle ships complete with aircraft and other emergency equipment. This is humanity in action, the kind of action expected of a compassionate and civilised world.

HIV/AIDS, on the other hand, was less dramatic, but many times more devastating than the tsunami. Yet it took over ten years of non-stop suffering and over twenty million deaths before the world started to act in some sort of meaningful way. When in early 2003, $15 billion was announced by President Bush it was appropriately called the "AIDS Emergency Relief Fund." Had the USA just woken up to the AIDS state of emergency? It had surely not just materialised overnight. Some of us had for years been crying our voices hoarse for help but it just fell on deaf ears.

Africa Pays with Blood

In March 2000, the Rockefeller Foundation facilitated me to carry out an in-depth study of the AIDS situation, focusing on East and Central Africa. This initiative was a brainchild of Dr. Florence Musiime who then worked with the Rockefeller Foundation equity section. She was supported in advancing her vision by her remarkable colleagues, especially Drs Tim Evans and Arial Peblos-Mendez among others, who, despite being non-Africans, clearly understood the imperative need for such a crucial study. They agreed with Dr Musiime that their foundation had a moral obligation to respond to the appalling AIDS situation in Africa. It was hoped that this study would provide data and compelling evidence that would galvanise rich countries and donors to come to the aid of Africa. Also commissioned were my proficient colleagues, Professor Suleymane M'boup from Senegal, who studied the West African situation, and Professor Ahmed Latif, a Zimbabwean, who took on the burning Southern Africa region. This project was an urgent effort to quickly document the magnitude of the AIDS problem, identify gaps and priorities including best practices in prevention, care and treatment, in order to inform an appropriate scientific response.

By the year 2000, the entire Sub–Saharan countries, with the exception of a few in West Africa, had established high levels of HIV, which were still on the rise. According to a UNAIDS report of June 2000, it was estimated that 5.4 million people worldwide became newly infected with HIV in 1999 alone. About 90% of these new infections were in the developing countries, particularly Sub-Saharan Africa. All these were in the pipeline of death to add to a staggering twenty-five million then already infected. That this was 70% of the world's disease burden and yet Africa had only 10% of the world's population underscored the magnitude of the tragedy.

Not unexpectedly, we found that AIDS was not only a devastating health and socio-economic problem, but it had also impacted disastrously on individuals, households, the community, governments and the region as a whole. Worse, it was still on a steep rise in almost all countries in Sub-Saharan Africa. Africa's hospital beds were overwhelmed with dying AIDS patients, some sharing beds while others filled the space on the floors and corridors. Meanwhile, over and above the catastrophe of AIDS, other serious endemic tropical diseases relentlessly massacred both the HIV infected and uninfected alike. In addition, an AIDS-fuelled Tuberculosis epidemic, shadowed by a steep rise in other opportunistic infections, was also wreaking havoc of its own. As AIDS annihilated the adults of childbearing age, the numbers of orphans mounted. In addition, the growing number of helpless orphans constituted a heavy burden on poor communities and posed a severe challenge to governments in the region.

The governments' meagre health expenditure was diverted to AIDS, without making any impact whatsoever because it was only being used to treat some of the symptoms but not the disease and its prevention. It was as if the paltry resources were just being poured down the drain. As a result, mortality rates skyrocketed and life expectancy nose-dived. The hard-won gains that had been achieved in the survival rates of children under five were being reversed. For instance, it was estimated by UNAIDS that Kenya would achieve a projected infant mortality rate of under fifty per 1000 thousand births by the year 2010, but because of AIDS alone the rates would more than reflect a doubling of the deaths. Other countries, including Malawi, Tanzania, Zambia and Zimbabwe, were projected with much worse predictions. In fact, in a publication on Wednesday June 28, 2000, headlined "AIDS SET TO DECIMATE NAMIBIAN POPULATION" it was reported "AIDS would claim the lives of half of all fifteen year olds in Namibia." This quoted an authoritative UNAIDS report that was released in Geneva, the previous day.

We also found that the huge numbers of AIDS patients and of those dying daily had far-reaching effects on the already very miserable lives of the people. AIDS had reversed many meaningful developments that had been achieved in Sub-Saharan Africa since independence. The governments and the many donor funded non-governmental organisations (NGOs) working in various fields and capacities were inundated, and some of them overwhelmed. Most organisations working in the field were uncoordinated in their activities, mainly due to their donors' all fingers and thumbs agendas. By and large, almost all of them concentrated their efforts on the easy options, thus limiting their impact on the ever worsening and challenging HIV/AIDS situation. At the very best, and however well intentioned, most donor projects were just scratching the surface.

Other findings as they emerged, though not entirely unexpected, were shocking even to us who lived with the catastrophe of AIDS daily. Simply put, the continent of Africa was ablaze with an out of control marauding killer disease that was shattering all aspects of life especially in Sub-Saharan Africa. All this mayhem was going on while the urgent cry for humanitarian relief had reached a crescendo, yet the rich countries and international organisations turned a deaf ear. All that was prescribed for the disaster was cheap but poorly funded, and thus non-effective; interventions such as information on prevention and Cotrimoxazole only. Africa was in the greatest need of the worldwide mobilisation of massive resources to help it cope with a catastrophe of unprecedented and unimaginable proportions, yet the world looked the other way.

It was apparent that in a continent where huge numbers of people were already infected, a preventive-only strategy could not possibly succeed unless it went hand in hand with a robust treatment programme. Prevention alone was like putting out the fire in a valley, while fuel flowed down the mountain. It was clear that Africa was in desperate need of the life-saving ART. We ascertained that the main constraint to ART access was the exorbitant cost of the drugs. It was apparent to us that the excuses of infrastructure deficiencies, lack of human resources and an ignorant population were mere apologies for the denial of a lifeline to poor people. In fact, all these so-called constraints, as we already knew, could be overcome in virtually all countries so paving the way for a quick scaling up of the life-saving therapy to the dying continent. Yet the pharmaceutical companies and their supporters insisted on record profits, oblivious to the horrific death toll while taking cover under these discredited excuses. Since Africans could not possibly pay the price and were not being helped by the rich countries, they just paid with their blood. It was all they had.

The East and Central African region that I studied was hit first, and particularly hard, by the HIV/AIDS epidemic. Uganda was the epicentre of the HIV epidemic from the early 1980s, up to the first half of the 1990s, with the highest HIV prevalence in the African continent and the world. However, Uganda instituted strong preventive measures under focused leadership, and after a decade of non-stop devastation, the epidemic started showing signs of decline. Up to now people still debate and ask: how did Uganda do it? In my research, I could not pinpoint a single knockout factor or a switch of some sort that turned around the epidemic. It was a combination of factors and interventions that did the trick. Certainly the good leadership by President Museveni in fighting AIDS played a major role. His government encouraged discussion and communication about AIDS, and educated the masses about the cause as well as how to protect oneself. It also created a conducive atmosphere for partners including NGOs and Community Based Organisations (CBOs) to operate. All these turned Uganda into a multi-pronged battleground against AIDS.

What were the other leaders in the region doing in the meantime? Many were doing the infamous ostrich act – burying their heads in denial. To them AIDS was shameful, dirty and frightening. It was bad news. It was feared that it would frighten tourism and investment away, which these countries desperately needed for their survival. Some saw AIDS as a Ugandan problem, a failed state and associated it with the chaos that had characterised the country's post-independence history. But Uganda was not an island. Winston Churchill once described Uganda as the pearl of Africa and others like to call it the heart of Africa, because it is right there in the centre of the continent. It has open borders with five countries. On both sides of every one of these borders reside people of the same tribes, including close relatives. The colonial borders insensitively divided the African continent totally ignoring the nationalities, kingdoms and ethnic borders. As the borders were too porous to police from the towns where the administrations of the colonial governments were comfortably ensconced, the people just moved relatively freely across borders and continue to do so today. Therefore denial was just an exercise in futility as AIDS was just a time bomb, which predictably exploded setting off an AIDS tsunami across the entire Sub-Saharan Africa. Yet the spread did not seem to be from Uganda as evidenced by the different HIV outbreaks found in various regions of the continent. AIDS just seemed to materialise everywhere.

There were of course other factors that could further explain the turn around of the Uganda epidemic. The sheer horror of it, which Ugandans had a longer time than other countries to suffer and endure, made people more receptive to self-preservation messages. The survival instinct of "flee or fight." Ugandan's embraced both. The youths by and large fled from sex as evidenced by postponement of sexual debut of youths from about sixteen years for females to over eighteen years and promiscuity was reduced. Those who, despite the threat, still continued having sex, and they were many, resorted to condoms. Uganda, a country where condoms were almost unknown, started using them by the millions and often running out of stock. This basic instinctive "flee or fight" reaction got to be known in the AIDS prevention jargon as "behavioural change", though part of it was acquired from information education, and communication. Admittedly, as described elsewhere other factors, should be taken into account that almost all AIDS patients of the early 1980s had died by the mid-1990s, and the new generation growing up at the time of heightened awareness had lower HIV rates, contributed to the overall lowering of rates, but only to a limited extent. Meanwhile the countries that kept their populations in the darkness woke up to find the epidemic not only knocking rudely at their doors but also firmly entrenched in their midst. The HIV pandemic, being so highly dynamic and yet insidious, took advantage of failure to institute timely responses resulting in an epicentre shift. By the late 1990s the Southern African region had taken over from Uganda for the highest HIV rates.

The alarming situation could also be partly explained by peculiar social, economic and cultural factors. By the mid-1980s, almost all countries in East and Central Africa had reported cases of HIV/AIDS, and since then the situation overall continued to deteriorate mainly due to widespread civil unrest, internal wars, social disruption and adverse socio-economic conditions. The chaotic situation that persisted in many countries could still be masking an even more serious problem. In fact, much later, in March 2005, the predictions were still grim, forecasting up to eighty million African deaths due to AIDS by the year 2025.

AIDS brought to Uganda and Africa a cascade of events that shook every aspect of life to the foundations and introduced new cultural and behavioural trends that were rapidly being established as norms. In a small number of cases, I saw the marvel of the African extended family resulting in people making sacrifices to save their poor relatives' lives. The sheer horror of the impending death of a sister, brother, son or other loved one brought out the best of the traditional spirit of pulling together, or *harambee*, as it is known in Kenya, in the face of danger. As a result, many poor patients, who would have otherwise died, survived. Admittedly this was comparatively just a drop in the ocean in contrast to the huge numbers who just helplessly perished. I witnessed many heroic endeavours that involved remarkable self-denial and sacrifice, mostly by women. I saw many seeking out all amenable relatives and organising family meetings at which the outpouring of sympathy and the fear of a looming death would compel a number of them to part with their meagre funds as contribution for life-saving therapy for a relative. The emotional attachment to the loved ones was, put to a severe test however as the numbers in dire need kept building up - overwhelmingly.

Time after time I met with individuals or groups of relatives of very ill patients who promised to fund their therapy. I would request them to make a firm commitment to support the long-term treatment of their relative since the disease was life long. Uniformly they would swear never to let their relatives down. Some complained that it was rude to even consider the possibility that they could fail to support their relative in mortal danger. However, as soon as there was improvement, thanks to the wonderful combination antiretroviral therapy, and the immediate threat of death was lifted, they would drift back to their chores and routine, once more give priority to the many other competing demands of life, including putting dinner on the table and paying school fees for their own children. Supporting treatment of their more distant relative would take second place, gradually fading out of the order of urgent priorities and eventually stop altogether.

Without antiretroviral drugs, treatment for AIDS opportunistic infections was recommended as the only feasible remedy for Africa. Yet in reality it was also too expensive, besides being ineffective. Once the AIDS stage set in, such treatment was just like mopping the floor without turning off the tap. One day it would be malaria, next pneumonia, followed by some other ailments, then terminal tuberculosis, toxoplasmosis, meningitis, cancer or some other serious AIDS-induced illness. The opportunistic infections, especially Tuberculosis (TB), were the terminal killers of most AIDS patients. TB, fuelled by HIV, was to become such a serious problem that by 2005 it was killing one patient every fifteen seconds. Yet TB could not be controlled without controlling HIV, and vice versa.

The opportunity to present our findings occurred at a major international meeting held in Kampala, Uganda, April 18 to 20, 2001, under the theme "AIDS Care in Africa." It was by far the biggest get together of the international experts and stakeholders on AIDS that specifically focused on scaling up AIDS care in Africa, and related research. The participants included health-care providers, ministries of health representatives, foundations, donor agencies, policy makers, international organisations, activists, and people living with AIDS from all over the world. President Museveni was the guest of honour and a keynote speaker. The meeting that is now acknowledged as the foundation of antiretroviral therapy in Africa was hosted by my organisation, the Joint Clinical Research Centre, at the Sheraton Hotel. It was jointly co-sponsored by Rockefeller Foundation, UNAIDS, United States National Institutes of Health, and The Global Forum for Health Research.

In the very first session I was nominated by colleagues Prof Mboup and Prof Latif to present our research findings that were to be the focus of this august conference. In my presentation I outlined AIDS epidemic evolvement in Africa, the then status of the epidemic, the grossly inadequate national and international responses, the debilitating constraints, and also made general and specific recommendations.

Using graphs and maps I was able to demonstrate the extent of AIDS devastation across the Sub-Saharan African region. Basically the self-explanatory data showed a continuing steep rise of new cases especially in Southern Africa, parallel with a rising death toll. The South African situation in particular was projected to deteriorate and the GDP was projected to decline by 17% by the year 2010, corresponding to a gross loss of over 22 billion dollars. With graphic cartoons, I demonstrated the heavy burden of AIDS on Africa and contrasted it with the miserable international responses. This very serious problem in Africa was being addressed only with rather vague preventive strategies that were generally ineffectual. Top among the gaps that we identified was the virtual absence of antiretroviral drugs, yet they were the craving of the over 25 millions Africans then estimated to be infected with HIV. The need was, of course, most acute among the over 3 million in immediate need of the life-saving drugs. Even the drugs for opportunistic infections that could have afforded AIDS patients some temporary relief were grossly deficient. In general terms the overall constraint that limited access to ARVs was poverty. I demonstrated that the huge numbers of AIDS patients and their poor governments just could not afford the exorbitantly-priced ARVs. In addition, all affected countries also had a huge debt burden. At the time AIDS treatment in Africa was still thought to be impossible and the funding requirements were frequently explained as a "bottomless pit." However, I was able to show that this was just unfortunate misinformation. I argued that ART was both a lifesaver and robust preventive tool. I explained that ART reduced mother to child HIV transmission, promoted voluntary counselling and testing, as people would be motivated to know their sero-status. It also reduced the general transmission of HIV, created better opportunities for surveillance, and stopped children from becoming orphans.

The conclusion of our landmark study, in a nut shell, was that: Africa was in urgent need of antiretroviral drugs side by side with a robust HIV preventive programme to curtail the AIDS carnage. This sounds rather obvious now, and to me it has always been so, but at the time it was widely propagated that Africa could not handle antiretroviral therapy and that only prevention was possible. Our study for the first time provided strong scientific data to counter the misinformation. Therefore, top among the recommendations emerging from our in-depth study was the clearly demonstrable urgent need for both antiretroviral therapy and robust prevention, and not just one without the other. Specifically there was need for international emergency help to save the continent from the abyss. There was palpable need for affordable ARVs, including cheaper generic drugs, as well as user-friendly and affordable monitoring tests. Accordingly, I called for urgent access to ARVs for Africa. I dismissed the myth that antiretroviral therapy could not be used in Africa. On the contrary I predicted that Africa would inevitably become the biggest user of ARVs in the world since the disease was most rampant on the continent. Many were moved by clear evidence that AIDS treatment was indeed imperative in Africa. Later at the farewell dinner, some participants confessed that they had not realised that AIDS was such a disaster in Africa. Medical journalists who attended the meeting, including one from the British Medical Journal, propagated our call for urgent access to ARVs and helped swell the international tide in support of AIDS care in Africa.

Among the participant at this crucial meeting was Dr Anthony Fauci of the United States National Institute of Health (NIH) on his first visit to Uganda. After the meeting he visited Rakai, the first Africa AIDS epicentre, and the JCRC, Africa's pioneer AIDS research centre. Dr Fauci was later to play a major role in advocating for funds for AIDS treatment from the US government, and was instrumental in the subsequent breakthrough.

Tragic Denial

While trying to increase access to AIDS drugs in Uganda, I met a number of so-called experts, including some I suspected to be proxies of business interests on apparent disinformation missions. I was especially incensed by their hackneyed utterances, like "incapacity of Africa to use antiretroviral therapy (ART)," because I had been successfully providing antiretroviral drugs to patients in Uganda since 1992. I used the same drugs as in the West with comparable outcome to the Western patients and, in some cases, even better. In my practice I had never encountered any special clinical difficulty other than the problem of the drugs' affordability. In fact, I often found, to my consternation, that some of the so-called authorities on ART had actually treated far fewer patients than I had. Pointing out this reality I would be met with disbelief, but fortunately our centre had collaborative relationships with external institutions and scientists who were able to independently confirm the facts. However, you just could not win them all over. Some doubting Thomases would still take it that if ART was being used, it would be our Western partners who were actually doing it for us. Not surprisingly, after so much propaganda, many people including some of the African doctors, believed that ART was too cumbersome to use in Africa. Likewise, in a publication by a South African judge in 2000, he supposed that it was only South Africa that was technically advanced enough to undertake the institutional use of ART in Africa.

Admittedly, it was quite cumbersome to start ART service in Uganda in the early 1990s, because of the exorbitant cost of the drugs. To complicate matters further, the pharmaceutical companies did not formally market their products in Africa as it was not lucrative. When I explained our plight to one American research collaborator working with us at the JCRC, he agreed to request his institution to allow us to buy the drugs from them and also to help with the shipment. We raised the seed money to pay for a small consignment of drugs and provided it at cost recovery to the small number of Ugandans able to afford it. This made it possible for us to make an early start and build up the necessary experience. In so doing we saved some lives that would have otherwise perished. In addition we also saved the relatively well off Ugandans the cost of the journeys to Europe where they used to go for the same treatment. To further increase access I adopted a policy of drugs market intelligence surveillance aimed at continuous identification of sources of cheaper but good quality drugs, which helped to increase the numbers of patients on therapy. However, the numbers accessing therapy remained small compared to the huge demand.

Back in 1993, there was much despondency in scientific circles all over the world because all the drugs being used for AIDS treatment were failing after a brief period of improvement, the exorbitant cost notwithstanding. In fact, it was openly stated by some scientists that long term effective AIDS treatment was just not possible. However, when the breakthrough in the form of effective combination antiretroviral drugs came in 1995 it came with such a prohibitive price tag that for the vast majority of Ugandans the drugs were as good as non-existent.

Perhaps the only country in Africa that had the economic muscle and expertise to dare use the newly discovered ART was South Africa, which by mid-1990s was facing the most catastrophic disaster due to AIDS. Incomprehensibly, it failed to take timely action to save its numerous citizens. Instead, the leadership curled into shameful denial, while hundreds of thousands died. Yet it was well within their stride to save them. Denial was led by no other than their otherwise great leaders who should have known better. What followed were some unfortunate decisions, including official hosting of some dubious scientific dissidents who engaged in a series of futile debates ostensibly to determine whether AIDS was caused by the HIV virus or not, whether antiretroviral drugs were effective, whether HIV was sexually transmitted and such other issues. If there had been any genuine doubt it would have been understandable to seek the best scientific guidance, to inform the fastest and most effective way forward. Yet most astoundingly, bonfide scientists were ignored and non-conformists and denialists were invited instead, allegedly to widen the scope of debate and ensure a variety of views. Yet AIDS was a catastrophic emergency. Some quacks from outside the continent, among them those who had never treated AIDS patients, joined in the debate on matters they either knew nothing about or chose to distort for their own agenda.

The situation was getting worse by the day, and by 2003 the World Bank's forecast for South Africa warned of possible economic decline/ collapse. The human toll was even more shocking. There were then about 4,500,000 people living with AIDS, of which an estimated 500 were dying daily. The country, usually full of lively, vibrant people was turning into a funeral republic. South Africa was evidently "on fire" yet incredibly a futile debate was raging, mainly concerning issues which had long been resolved scientifically. Inaction was very tragic in terms of the human and economic toll. There was a misconception that antiretroviral drugs were too toxic and too expensive. Try death instead? In reality, if the total cost of other interventions without ART were put in monetory terms, it would have been found to be shockingly high, human suffering notwithstanding. Incredibly, a proven solution, namely ART, known to be feasible and highly effective, was ignored.

Eventually the outcry could no longer be ignored, and South Africa eventually took a belated action, though too little, and too late for the millions dead and others still destined to die. A treatment target of just over 50,000 to be on ART by May 2005 was set up by the government. This was far too low for Africa's richest country, with the world's biggest numbers of AIDS patients, who had by then risen to about 5,000,000 infected and at least 450,000 of them in immediate need of the lifesaving drugs. When I attended an AIDS workshop in Bloemfontein, South Africa, on March, 30,2005, I was stunned to learn that even this small number was not going to be reached. I asked a few "experts" at the meeting why it was that South Africa could not treat this small number of patients. One apologist started telling me how complicated ART therapy was! South Africa is Africa's medical flagship and patients from all over the continent in need of sophisticated medical care, including many Ugandans, flock there daily. The country has some of the continent's best experts and the most sophisticated medical facilities. It carried out the world's first heart transplant and boasts a world-class infrastructure, although admittedly also some of the worst. Yet here was this so-called expert telling me that the country was incapable of treating desperately ill patients with relatively simple drugs, which in generic form consisted of just one pill to be taken by a patient twice daily. I could not believe what I was hearing! At the Bloemfontein meeting a South African pharmaceutical company, Aspen, displayed quality generic AIDS drugs produced in South Africa. When I asked them whether they had drugs in stock, they confirmed that not only did they have a lot in stock, but also were able to increase production to meet increased demand. Yet over an estimated 500 people were dying daily. Dying of a mainly preventable death.

A little earlier in 2000, as South Africa belatedly started preparing to use low-cost generic ART that had recently become available, the brand manufacturers took the country to court. The drug companies looked like insensitive profiteers as they braved massive protests, which built up around the courthouse in Pretoria. The world's television aired the shocking pictures of blatant greed, and the drugs companies' corporate image suffered. This kind of case could not have been brought against a powerful country like the USA or Canada. When there was a much smaller threat of Anthrax, though never expected to reach the scale of the AIDS disaster, no nonsense about the patents of a life-saving drug (Ciprofloxacin) was entertained while American and Canadian lives were at stake. Canada made it clear that it would use generics if the need arose. However, as expected, the patent holder quickly consented to US demands to make the drug immediately affordable for what turned out to be a non-existent public emergency.

Indirectly the South African inaction and denial was partly responsible for the lawsuit. The country had not clearly declared AIDS a national disaster, and any indirect references to it were muted. At the very least, the government's actions were not the frantic response commensurate with the magnitude of the scourge. Yet the demands for therapy had reached a crescendo not only in South Africa but Africa as a whole. It was clear that a violation of human rights was being committed against the poor of the world. The silver lining to this big Pharma debacle and the South African government inaction was that it highlighted to the world the carnage of AIDS in Africa as a moral imperative. No one could deny it any more: it was ethically and morally unacceptable to let so many die by deliberate denial even if international treaties condoned it.

The Moral Imperative

By 1999 the AIDS epidemic in Sub-Saharan Africa was still expanding, mirrored by the increasing death toll. According to UNAIDS release, the year saw 2.6 millions worldwide deaths from HIV/AIDS, the highest since the beginning of the epidemic. The overwhelming numbers of the deaths were in Africa, and mostly among those aged below 40 years of age. Evidently, the carnage and sheer horror of the situation could not be ignored any more. The rich world was increasingly finding it just morally unacceptable to continue sitting idly by unsympathetically watching the annihilation of the poor and the wretched of the earth, when it was within their powers and means to at least ameliorate the situation. They were also facing mounting criticism from human rights organisations that accused their leaders of callous indifference in the face of a humanitarian crisis

In time worldwide protests spread, as activists decried the paucity of global action in the face of a catastrophe of this magnitude and, more especially, they demanded that antiretroviral therapy be made accessible to at least those whose lives were in immediate danger. They protested against the enforcement of TRIPS, and patent laws under which the pharmaceutical companies maintained monopoly rights for production, and the exorbitant pricing of ARVs. Without market competition that normally regulates prices, the life-saving AIDS drugs cost that would reverse the trend remained unaffordable to millions of dying Africans. Therefore the following year's death toll was already predicted to become more devastating and progressively bleak in subsequent years. Protest parades (often including peaceful people who never thought they would be involved in any street demonstrations), at least in one instance including Nelson Mandela, mushroomed in many capitals of the world. Placard-waving activists besieged pharmaceutical stalls at all AIDS conferences and held protests at the venues of all G8 meetings, turning them into fortresses. The hackneyed excuses of poor infrastructure, lack of human resources and poor or non-existent logistics in Africa for the deplorable inaction in the face of such a devastating humanitarian catastrophe was no longer tenable as justification.

This bleak period became a very busy time for me as I was constantly on the move to many parts of the world, to present scientific data illustrating the carnage of AIDS in Africa, and the urgent need for antiretroviral treatment. I aimed to counter the widespread misinformation that mass AIDS treatment was not possible in Africa. I presented an easy-to-implement model that we developed at the Joint Clinical Research Centre in Uganda, which was successfully applied to extend therapy to some rural areas. However, drugs access remained very limited because of affordability constraints. In almost all my presentations, I made it a point to include a PowerPoint slide that asked a question:

"IS ANTIRETROVIRAL FEASIBLE IN AFRICA?"

And the answer would follow in as large a bold red print as would fit the screen:

"YES!"

I always added that the only constraint was:

"THE EXORBITANT COST OF THE DRUGS"

And that all other constraints could be easily overcome.

I took this message to the USA, Europe, Asia, and the Caribbean - and to all meetings wherever I was invited. I made it a special mission to make sure that as many of my fellow Africans as I could reach got the message so that we could together keep up the pressure to bring about the desperately needed relief for our dying people.

However, millions of dollars invested in the misinformation machinery had done incredible damage to many people's view of the AIDS situation in Africa. Not surprisingly many remained unaware of the inside story of AIDS devastation. Hitherto, I still meet many who either do not believe it, or think that the sad events have somehow been deliberately exaggerated. Some people even think that there is an unfair campaign going on against the pharmaceutical companies. Yet, among those that were in position to know, are many apologists that would tell me that the whole debacle was nobody's fault and that, if anything, it was Africa herself to blame for her own suffering.

"The sophistication associated with antiretroviral therapy makes it impossible for its safe and effective use in Africa, because of her dismal infrastructure, illiterate populations, and deficiently qualified medical care providers," was almost like a hit song chorus of the time.

Addressing US Congress one prominent American expert said: "The drugs have to be taken on time. If say the drug needs to be taken at ten o'clock, the Africans will ask: what does ten o'clock mean?" He was, of course, trying to dissuade the US government from giving any money for the treatment of AIDS in Africa. I do not believe even for a moment that this good gentleman harboured any malicious intent against the Africans, especially as he was an African-American himself. It was more likely that he was merely a victim of misinformation. The entire misinformation machinery aimed at protecting the money-spinning AIDS drugs monopoly had the powerful world decision-makers as prime targets.

However, I too got an opportunity to testify to the US Senate, and while I prepared my presentation, one prominent American AIDS researcher asked to see my presentation in advance. I obliged because I wanted all the possible support and advice in making a powerful presentation that had to succeed for all humanity's sake. However, when she read through the draft, she immediately saw red, and sent me an SOS.

"Drop any reference to antiretroviral drugs," she pleaded. "To the conservatives in the US Senate, any reference to antiretroviral drugs is sure to kill any help for Africa!"

I was, however, not ready to compromise on this issue. Antiretroviral therapy was, as far as I was concerned, the very crux of the matter. I was not at all prepared to settle for the usual tokens normally prescribed for Africa, which in practice did not make any difference. I was determined to tell them what was really required and firmly reject meaningless gestures. After all, there was nothing to lose since there was no serious donation ongoing or in the pipeline for AIDS relief in Africa. There were too many token AIDS projects in Africa mainly to do with Voluntary Counselling and Testing, even then on a very small scale, whose net effect was minimal. The only intervention that would put a stop to the massive number of deaths was antiretroviral therapy. Therefore, I was resolute that I was going to request the Senate for antiretroviral therapy and not some diversionary non-consequential interventions. However, she had read the mood of the US Senate correctly, in that only the easy options for Africa stood a good chance of attracting some funding support from the West, as I was to find out later.

On April 11, 2001, I testified to the US Senate committee on *Health Education Labour and Pensions: capacity to care in a world living with AIDS,* chaired by Senator Edward Kennedy. The other senators present were Hillary Clinton, Patty Murray, and Christopher Dodd (all Democrats) and Senator Bill Frist, John Warner and Jeff Sessions, the Republicans. Frist had recently been on a visit to Uganda that included the JCRC, where I took the opportunity to make a special presentation to him about our work that clearly demonstrated that we had the capacity to treat AIDS if we had the necessary resources. He therefore knew first hand the devastating effect of HIV/AIDS on individual patients and their families in Uganda. As a doctor himself, he was in a unique position to understand and appreciate the urgent need for AIDS therapy. I was therefore gratified that he was among the senators listening to the testimony. Hillary Clinton too had recently been on a tour of Uganda where she too saw the devastation of AIDS. Therefore I had good reason to expect that this particular US Senate sub-committee would make a difference.

In my presentation, I talked about the devastation of AIDS in Africa, the exorbitant cost of AIDS drugs and the most urgent and critical need for the life-saving treatment. During question time I deplored the exorbitant cost of drugs and tests. At the time the cost of both CD4 and Viral Load was a staggering $200, equivalent to five months' salary of a Ugandan primary school teacher. In my presentation, I hoped that the focus would remain firmly on the real reason why millions of people were dying in Africa, which was first and foremost the shameful denial of life saving treatment. However, when it came to question time, I was taken aback when Senator Frist, of all people, appeared to ignore the real killer that he had seen with his own eyes, and instead chose to ask me about the cost of the AIDS test. Alarm bells rang in my head. It was back to the usual token gestures again.

Besides the JCRC, I figured that during his brief visit to Uganda Senator Frist would have been taken around to see a few US-funded AIDS projects in Uganda that included an AIDS testing centre. I imagined that as usual the US technocrats would have taken the opportunity to exaggerate the role US government played in the alleviation of AIDS in Uganda by projecting the AIDS testing support as a big humanitarian contribution. Yet the reality on the ground was that the US funding to Uganda and Africa at large addressed only the easiest and cheapest options, which did not offer any relief to the millions of AIDS patients, and did not have any substantial impact on the epidemic. For instance, the much-hyped financial support for HIV tests that the US funded through USAID was initially free because only a small number of people volunteered for testing. When the numbers increased slightly a cost-sharing price tag of about a dollar per person was introduced, without any other follow-up intervention. That left all those who tested positive in dead end. The only option open to them was to prepare for a painful death since treatment was neither funded nor affordable.

I had counted so much on the support of Senator Frist for treatment funding since I had made an impassioned presentation pleading for AIDS treatment during his Uganda visit, and personally showed him the soon-to-die patients in desperate need. I felt let down, and disappointed that the support I expected from him did not materialise. Worse still, I was troubled that by asking a question about the cost of AIDS test, Frist was trying to divert attention from our most critical need by throwing a hint to his colleagues that AIDS testing was the way to go. And who would doubt him since he had personally visited Africa to see what needed to be done there? That question dimmed any hope that something serious would come out of this meeting. The overwhelming outcry of our dying people was for antiretroviral therapy. AIDS testing was the very first and only significant project that the US had funded in Uganda from the late 1980s. Many people were understandably reluctant to volunteer for AIDS testing because without treatment they could see only worry and doom. Yet here we were over a decade later, in the US Senate, listening to the same old question and a tip-off that it was all that Africa could expect. It was not that I thought testing was not necessary, but I wanted it clearly understood that the state of the AIDS crisis in Africa called for nothing short of massive and meaningful interventions that would make a real difference and not merely the usual one dollar cheap token projects that did not address the epidemic.

I was also asked to comment on the military and security implication of AIDS. I explained that AIDS was a serious destabilising factor in Africa. AIDS without treatment and good morale in the military do not go hand in hand. Obviously, soldiers weakened by AIDS could not be expected to defend their country and keep the peace. The increasing agitation for therapy and desperation made AIDS a volatile political issue in Africa.

The most memorable part for many participants of the April 11, 2001 Senate hearing was not AIDS however. The show was stolen by one of my fellow contributors. He was none other than Sir Elton John. He attracted much attention. Some dignitaries, including senators, turned up excitedly to see him. I watched with amusement as some senators and dignitaries turned up with their Elton John records for autographs and a rare opportunity to pose for a picture with him. His presence appeared to be much more important than his message against AIDS, but at least it pulled in the crowds.

The overall impression I got from the Senate meeting was that while we succeeded in getting the senators to listen to our pleas for help, we still failed to change their preconceived opinions. We, made it clear however, that AIDS in Africa was a moral imperative, necessitating urgent action. The Senate was then under the control of Democrats who are traditionally thought of as natural allies of the poor, the minorities and the developing countries, rather than Republicans. Yet, according to my humble observations, at least with regard to Global AIDS, they hardly ever demonstrate it in actions. In fact, they committedonly little money for the urgently needed treatment of AIDS. Ironically, the breakthrough was to come later when the Republicans took over control of the Senate. I was also involved in this exercise with the Republicans and saw a different approach as described later. As a non-American, it is difficult for me to make out the intricacies of American politics. However, on a superficial assessment, it looks to me like the Democrats tend to procrastinate making any substantial commitment to Third World countries or their poor minorities because they seem to suffer from some sort of stigma - a fear of being labelled "spendthrift liberals" - while the Republicans, on the other hand appear to be much more decisive on causes that somehow coincide with or serve their agenda.

Continuing my crusade, I always had a simple but powerful answer to those who for whatever reason gave the excuse that antiretroviral therapy was simply impossible in Africa: "We are doing it in Uganda," I would say to them. Initially this used to be received with disbelief, despite my clear data and illustrations. Yet the JCRC had used antiretroviral drugs since 1991, starting with AZT, which was the first to become available, and went on to introduce follow-on drugs as they became available. I would keep insisting that the price of drugs was the only constraint that we had encountered in our otherwise successful treatment programme. It was the cost which limited access to a very tiny minority of our people. I emphasised that the most important intervention essential for saving lives and with the power to put a stop to the agony of dying AIDS patients in Africa was affordable drugs. I repeatedly called upon our experience at the JCRC and our scale up model to demonstrate that virtually all other constraints could be overcome. However, despite the data and facts clearly demonstrating a way forward across Sub-Saharan Africa, some hard-core profiteers and apologists put up a spirited resistance. They often resorted to diversionary and scare tactics warning of dire consequences including widespread drugs resistance if AIDS drugs were, as it was frequently put, "parachuted" into Africa, as justification for their money spinning business as usual.

Meanwhile, in developed and rich industrialised countries, AIDS had long ceased to be a major public health problem except in special risk groups. Great scientific advances had been achieved in the areas of prevention and treatment. Indeed, morbidity and mortality from HIV infection had dramatically declined. ART had made mother-to-child transmission so rare as to be almost non-existent. Yet, these impressive advances had not reached Africa where the need was most acute and the problem most serious. There was therefore a rising outrage, a moral dilemma and a new sense of urgency in both the local and international arena demanding humanitarian redress of this extreme and unethical situation. It was no longer tenable to sit on the fence while millions perished. It was also becoming very uncomfortable even to the pharmaceutical companies to continue reaping huge profits while AIDS committed genocide, as if it was the Middle Ages. However, the situation in the Middle Ages was different and excusable, because treatments for infectious diseases of the time were unknown.

4

Dubious Schemes

Do Patents Really Kill?

Robert Guest wrote an intriguing book, *The Shackled Continent,* which by definition and the historical perspectives of her people could only be Africa. In it, he described so much that is wrong with the continent, including mind-boggling chaos, incompetence, corruption, nepotism, mistrust, treachery, dreadful systems and bad governance. One cannot help but mostly agree with Guest as he recounts stories of some shameful African regimes that killed and plundered Africa's wealth and reversed any achievements that they found in place when they ascended to, or as was more often the case, grabbed power. A quick roll call of Africa's leaders now would show that despite some progress in a few areas, the situation still remains dire. Guest, like many other Westerners who take an interest in Africa, no matter the purpose, went as far as prescribing some remedies. Undeniably, many of Guest's findings are true, though at times his diagnosis and prescriptions are contentious.

However, he seems to have got the wrong end of the stick with regard to one crucial issue - namely AIDS drugs access in Africa. This was in reference to the scandalous denial of life-saving AIDS drugs to millions of Africans who had died, and millions more in the pipeline - doomed to perish en masse from a preventable death. He asserted that pharmaceutical companies need protection by patents law, so that they could have strong incentives to innovate new drugs. In effect, this implies that it is justifiable for the pharmaceutical companies to charge exorbitant prices and make huge profits from life-saving drugs, totally oblivious to the plight of the poor, even if millions died an awful death. His rationalisation was that the drugs' discovery and development into finished pharmaceutical products cost a huge amount of money, which the companies needed to recoup. This is the song that pharmaceutical companies have sung all along, and would very much like everybody to believe. In fact, they have spent a fortune to get this point hammered into as many influential people's brains as possible. The truth is that pharmaceutical companies have never had a priority agenda to rush in to help disease-ridden, poor African countries. They certainly did not exude any great enthusiasm to act in a hurry or change their practice in the face of the magnitude of the AIDS catastrophe.

As described earlier, at least one drug Zidovudine (AZT) that hitherto remains one of the constituents of Highly Active Antiretroviral Therapy (HAART) was discovered long before the era of AIDS. It was not specifically discovered for the treatment of AIDS, yet it reaped the lion's share of an unprecedented fortune, initially for its foster parent *Burroughs Wellcome*, and then for the inheritors of the company. The history of AZT exposes the bluff of those who vainly try to justify the denial of therapy to millions on the basis of recouping big investments incurred during the discovery of AIDS drugs. In reality, it was Jerome Horowitz who was the true discoverer of AZT and he did so long before the era of HIV/AIDS, back in 1964, when he worked for the National Cancer Institute of the USA. AZT was discovered as a candidate cancer drug. However, it flopped, and thereafter just remained on the shelf, unwanted by any pharmaceutical company as an "orphan drug." This was until the onset of AIDS when virtually everything at hand was being frantically tested for antiviral activity. In 1985 AZT was among the drugs that were randomly picked for testing and by luck was found to have an effect on HIV. Therefore, this later re-discovery of AZT in its new role as an AIDS drug was not exactly an act of scientific genius. It was approved in close to record time in 1987 as a pioneer antiretroviral drug. Yet a company that had nothing to do with its original discovery, *Wellcome,* marketed AZT as an innovative, highflying, high tech, and very expensive drug. The more money a drug makes, the more the law, irrespective of other factors, protects it. The patents protection in the case of AZT, as in many other cases of highly lucrative drugs, had little to do with intellectual property rights. It had more to do with profits.

In 1992, the year I was frantically looking for an alternative therapy for our poor patients, it was reported that a massive 44.7 tones of AZT produced that year returned *Wellcome* over £250 million in profit! Ironically this might have been the only time in this tragic story that our poor African patients were lucky to be denied access to therapy, since they actually lost nothing. First of all, the effect of AZT as a single drug treatment for AIDS was only transient, since the virus quickly developed resistance to it. Secondly, the high drug dosages used at that time were very toxic, often causing life threatening or lethal side effects. Yet, at the end of the day, it had no significant durable survival benefit.

A number of follow-on drugs of the same general class were discovered merely by chemical engineering of the same old Zidovudine molecule. In fact, some important drugs were developed with US public money, yet the pharmaceutical companies that stepped in to commercially exploit the discovery never made allowances for this vital contribution by the public. Furthermore, the pharmaceutical companies are required by law to provide accurate accounts of costs in their tax returns. The declared amounts spent in the development of drugs to which they would be entitled to claim tax exemption do not always tally with the purportedly huge amount of money spent in the development of the drugs. Therefore, the assertion that pharmaceutical companies are forced to hike the drugs costs because of the research investments does not always hold water.

Nevertheless, it would be naïve to deny that the pharmaceutical industry spends huge amounts of money in drugs' development. If that had been the case, it would not be the undisputed world's most powerful and influential industry. By 2002 it was estimated that the industry was investing to the tune of a staggering $27 billion per year in new drugs research. However, this was by and large for profit-targeted products for the lucrative Western markets, mainly lifestyle drugs like those for impotence, hair growth, or common Western conditions like cholesterol, depression, and obesity. Lifestyle drugs are protected the same way as emergency and life saving drugs, irrespective of whether they are critically needed by the poor to avert massive deaths.

In 1998, WHO funded some researchers to try and find out why tuberculosis (TB) drugs were not being manufactured by the big

Pharma. A parallel AIDS-fuelled TB epidemic is on the rampage in the same countries devastated by AIDS. Predictably, the researchers found that market demand was more than or just as important as science in guiding the decision of pharmaceutical companies. "The major companies are aiming for $1 billion at peak sales," the study concluded. When this is the target you certainly do not look to Africa where that kind of money exists only in Sunday afternoon siesta dreams! In another widely quoted study led by Dr Bernard Pecoul, it was found that of the 1,233 drugs patented between 1975 and 1997, only thirteen were for tropical diseases. Before hastening to thank the pharmaceutical companies for this small favour, pause to scrutinise the nature of the thirteen drugs: a mere four were for human tropical diseases. Some of the other nine came from work by the USA army specifically for the Vietnam War targeting diseases that might affect their soldiers. Others were from research on drugs for livestock or for the pet market, which was colourfully described as a "potential gold mine."

Meanwhile more important diseases devastating the poor were just ignored. These include devastating killer tropical diseases like Trypanosomiasis, more commonly known as Sleeping Sickness. This painful killer disease is marauding across Central and Eastern Africa with mainly two ancient highly toxic drugs of the 1920s, including Melarsoprol, as the only ones available to treat it. Worse still, a resistant type of Sleeping Sickness is spreading and yet an alternative drug effective against it was abandoned by its manufacturer. This was Eflornithine, dubbed the "Resurrection drug" because it brought back to life people in coma who had been given up for dead. It was just dropped like a hot potato once it was clear it would not make money. The manufacturer was not even interested in the patent, for which they would otherwise almost lay down their lives to protect, simply because poor Sleeping Sickness sufferers did not constitute a lucrative market. The drug was signed off absolutely free of charge to the WHO, which had a tough time finding a new manufacturer. In contrast, another drug, which could also be dubbed the resurrection drug, but in an entirely different context, is the old Pentamidine of the early 1940s which was only effective during the very early stages of Sleeping Sickness

- before the parasites enter the brain. The drug was, until early 1980s, of almost no interest to the pharmaceutical companies and was either given out free or just sold for a little amount. That was until its sudden resurrection following the discovery that it was a dormant gold mine. Its change of fortunes was triggered by the discovery that it was effective against a life threatening AIDS opportunistic infection, Pneumocystis Pneumonia (PCP), which at the time was raging among AIDS patients in the West. Then pharmaceutical companies' interest (read 'greed') returned. As a result the price shot up a stunning thirty times complete ,with a new trade name to go with it! The newly-repackaged version was, of course, not accessible to the poor, and the old stocks that were previously being given out freely just melted into thin air. Yet the same killer PCP was heading to Africa.

For a long time no major pharmaceutical company invested any significant amounts of funding in new research on therapies for Sleeping Sickness. Most scientists agree that the development of new drugs for this excruciatingly painful and fatal disease would be a priority if it affected any part of the West. It would certainly not be as difficult as, say, high tech drugs for treatment of dog separation anxiety or dog Alzheimer's disease. Modern drugs to help dogs not to "worry" too much or become too forgetful are available and made by the great Novartis and Pfizer respectively. Certainly no one would begrudge a "rich" dog its hard-earned comfort, or dispute the need to develop animal drugs but this puts the profit-driven priorities of the big Pharma in vivid perspective.

Sleeping Sickness, Leishmaniasis, Elephantiasis (otherwise known as Lymphatic Filiasis) and a number of other tropical diseases without modern drugs for their treatment are referred to as "orphan diseases". As far as the pharmaceutical world is concerned, it is almost always profits that motivate the development of new drugs. Many would understand if the profits were reasonable. The problem is the unwarranted exorbitant price. Additionally, the current patent protection period of twenty years per newly patented drug is agonisingly too long. This is especially painful as the drugs are the only ones available for the treatment of an excruciating killer disease - AIDS. Even when the patent has expired for a highly lucrative drug still in high demand, the patent holder often finds some loopholes to extend it by merely doing some minor alteration to the drug. This was done inthe case of Pentamidine to make it appear like it was different, thus extending the agony and suffering of those unable to access it. With regard to AIDS, there is no doubt that pharmaceutical companies have reaped huge profits out of this truly humanitarian tragedy, and had plenty to spare for propaganda purposes, and to denigrate anyone who challenges their excessive earnings.

Perhaps not surprisingly Mr. Guest and others take exception to the assertion by AIDS activists that "Patents kill!" Mr. Guest observed, "This is unfair." And added, "Without patents there would be no incentives for private companies to invent new medicines." Which medicines did Mr. Guest refer to? Certainly not the drugs for poor people's diseases. From a Sub-Saharan African perspective, and the poor Africans therein, the net effect of patents (though it was never spelt out as such) with regard to life threatening diseases like AIDS, is as if they were specifically targeted for genocide. Certainly not Rwanda- style - but by denial. This kind of death is not dramatic enough to make it into the *Breaking News*. It is a slow but sure killer. Most poor people just suffer silently or whimper quietly in pain until death, without loud screams to spoil the world's most lucrative business. Patents definitely contributed to the AIDS drugs being so exorbitantly priced, and for so long, and the big contributor to the massive AIDS death toll. Pursuit of profits is dictating the choice of drugs to make, and where to market them, and it is generally blind to the humanitarian considerations of the poor.

Nobody is in any doubt that AIDS has already massacred millions of Africans. Appallingly, this horror and mayhem was allowed to go on after effective therapy became available. The life-saving drugs could have been more readily and cheaply made available to the poor if generic manufacturers were not constrained by patents laws. There were many countries and industries able and ready to make AIDS drugs accessible to patients at a more affordable price. However, patent holders adamantly refused to allow this, and threatened with litigation some of those that tried to manufacture them cheaply and make them more widely available to a larger number of suffering people. They insisted on exacting their "legitimate" pound of flesh. Never mind that people suffered and died a horrific death in huge numbers. Through all this mayhem, the law to protect the pharmaceutical companies must be upheld. Otherwise, they threaten: "Kiss fare well to innovation and newer life-saving drugs." Yet the newer life-saving drugs never go to where the killer diseases are. They go where the money is.

In addition to rampant poverty, race, cultural and religious differences we need to put patents on the list of issues that need to be urgently addressed in order to make planet Earth a better place for humanity. We need new international laws that ensure humanity unreserved protection against killer diseases now and in future. Currently no one rich or poor prefers a system that prioritises profits far above public health. There is a need to get rid of any factors which give an excuse for the spread of radicalism among the deprived and marginalised, but otherwise good, peoples, of the world. Why then is this injustice passing largely unnoticed in the West where there are many more vocal humanitarian organisations than anywhere else with a capacity to fight it? Many Western humanitarian organisations flock to the poor countries to monitor everything ranging from government performances to sexual preferences, yet ignore what has turned out to be one of the most lethal human rights issues.

There appears to have been two major reasons why this injustice in not so explicit. First of all, the drugs manufacturers spend billions in lobby fees to ensure that they are perceived in a good light, while making sure that loopholes are blocked thus guaranteeing their unchallenged monopoly. There is also an ongoing disinformation campaign linked to wide advertisement of token, or what has been described by activists as "spurious", donor projects whose real worth to the poor is often highly exaggerated. All that many people in the West ever get to hear about the big Pharma with regard to their business with AIDS ridden poor African countries is "the huge cost reductions and generous donations" that they regularly announce in a hullabaloo of publicity. The sad reality, as described later, is that such gestures are not always what they appear to be.

Meanwhile, the ordinary people in the West do not always suffer the direct consequence of the exorbitant cost of drugs. This is due to the fact that their drugs are not paid for directly out of a patient's pocket, as is the case in poor countries. In the West insurance companies mainly pay for drugs. Woe to the one without insurance in USA and most of the West! He or she either suffers the same fate as a poor African or is just relegated to the mercy of charities. Therefore, the huge cost of drugs is not readily felt in the West, as is the case in poverty-stricken Africa. Insurance is almost unknown in many poor countries. It is ironic that the very poor are the very ones left to foot the huge cost of drugs directly out of their empty pockets.

Admittedly, not only the pharmaceutical companies are to blame for this sad situation. After all, they are not primarily humanitarian organisations though they often adopt this pose for promotional reasons. Asked to comment about this situation one Aventis spokesman, Mr Gros, is quoted as having said, 'The industry has never been philanthropic. It has always produced products with an aim to getting a return on investment." So who according to the big Pharma should be taking care of the interests of the poor people since pharmaceutical companies are basically "for-profit" organisations? Incredibly it is yet another Aventis spokesman, Mr Aumonier, who provided an insight into that issue, "Access to medicine is a human right." He pondered the aphorism frequently used by health activists. "I like that statement," he declared philosophically. "But it is a right that should be enforced by the whole community." Then he added, "May I suggest that the pharmaceutical industry is only part of that community?" Precisely! This is the very reason why humanitarian-friendly patent laws and trade rules need to be introduced because the world community, with the big Pharma inclusive, cannot condone a practice that leads to massive suffering and deaths in exchange for unregulated profits. But the philosopher had not yet finished. "What is to be done if the poor are too poor to buy drugs on the free market? Does government act sufficiently? To say to industry 'you make money, so you must enforce this human right alone' – this, somewhere is wrong." Here, of course, he means that governments should pay for the drugs. This possibility needs to be explored as well, and how it may be implemented. But currently getting paid is the beginning and end of pharmaceutical business. But at least Mr Aumonier acknowledged the dilemma. Humanity has cardinal rights that must be protected. Just like we had the Helsinki Declaration to address the holocaust and other violations of human rights, like the Tuskegee human experiments, we also need ethical rules to govern use and accessibility to life-saving drugs for humanity's sake. This needs a solution at global level, with active involvement of the West working with the poor countries in good faith to get the world governments together to put a stop to the carnage, through enactment of better and straight TRIPS and patents laws. If the present laws - as vividly illustrated by the devastation and anguish they have caused to AIDS victims - are not seen as gross human rights violation now, then certainly future generations will look back in shock and disbelief. At the very least they will wonder how this gross violation of human rights was allowed to happen.

Surely there must be a more humanitarian and ethical alternative to the current practice. If TRIPS (Trade Related aspects of Intellectual Property Rights) and patents laws were so good and do not really kill, as some claim, then what explanation should be given to the relatives, friends and fellow citizens of the millions of people who perished simply because life-saving drugs were denied them on account of their poverty?

Just for a moment, imagine that we live in a world where only the rich had access to drugs for a treatable mass killer disease. Then stop imagining – because it is real and it is legal! It is also real that the same patent law which protects against copying an innovative device developed to alert a dog that its master is approaching, is protected and applied in exactly the same way to life saving medicines - including critical drugs to stop mass deaths, or a tragic humanitarian emergency like bio-terrorism.

Patents law in its present would not be as painful if the gap between the "haves and the have-nots" of the world was not so wide. In terms of the carnage and human suffering, gross violations of human rights could have been committed from the mid-1990s when effective therapies for AIDS finally became available. Yet for almost a decade no serious action was taken to rush these newly-discovered drugs to Africa to put a stop to the carnage. On the contrary, the rules that denied access to the life-saving therapy were enforced. While it all happened the rich world watched seemingly in limbo, occasionally uttering some apologetic excuses. Meanwhile drugs companies continued as usual, totally oblivious to the plight of the huge numbers of poor people who were left to die excruciatingly. I submit that future generations may rank this among the candidates for one of the biggest violations of human rights in history. At least the incomparable holocaust did not have any international laws to back up the crimes. The perpetuators of the holocaust have been hounded down and, whenever caught, they are swiftly brought to justice. On the contrary no one has specifically broken any current law in the matter of the deaths of millions by the denial of AIDS life-saving drugs on account of their (poverty) failure to pay the price. It is all "perfectly" lawful.

In all fairness, not all blame should be put on the shoulders of the rich countries, but also to some extent on the African countries themselves. I strongly feel that it is not beyond the means of any country to, at least, throw a bucket of water into the towering inferno that was raging on the continent. Africans and their leaders should have been in the forefront of highlighting their own plight by creating worldwide awareness about the carnage on the continent. Unfortunately, most African leaders were engrossed in other chronic and recurrent crises on the continent. Yet it was AIDS that was the most serious by far. African activists who manage to get any publicity are usually European or American-based and in some cases are detached from the day-to-day realities in Africa. I have witnessed with utter resignation some Africans taking up activism not for purposes of making a difference but rather as a livelihood. A number of them are poor and poorly educated with a shallow grasp of the pertinent issues, and thus end up inadvertently sabotaging serious efforts to redress the injustice confronting Africa through their unawareness of the salient issues. Poverty did not mean that African governments had absolutely no funds. After all, the scourge was killing our own citizens in huge numbers under our very noses. Where was our wrath?

African leaders could at least have declared a continent-wide state of emergency. They could have lobbied the world as a unitary body highlighting the fact that the continent was in mortal danger. Resources, however meagre, could have been mobilised. Although the amounts would have fallen short of the required sum, such an initiative would have formed the best basis for a bargaining position. They could have negotiated effectively and in unison for lower cost generics drugs, and allocated some funds, however modest, so that they could immediately start saving as many lives as possible on their own initiative while they asked for help. They could have used their very best brains side by side with politicians, to form a proficient team to present to the WTO a strong united African appeal and proposal for the urgent revision of TRIPS and patents laws. There are, of course, lots more that African countries could have done, but did not do. Sadly some were paralysed by stigma, others by corruption, colonial hangovers, and incompetence, or else were just overwhelmed by the sheer magnitude of the problem and the formidable odds against them. While their inaction could not be condoned, it does not in any way justify the shameful international failure to come to the aid of Africa faced with such a devastating emergency humanitarian calamity.

Giving a Rope to the Poor

AIDS carnage to date rivals that of the horrific so-called Black Death and will, at the continuing current rate of carnage, surpass it before this pandemic is through. Forty million more lives and still rising, equivalent to the entire populations of about half a dozen small African nations, are at stake. The vast majority of AIDS sufferers are in Africa, yet the continent is without the resources to cope with such a massive disaster.

To insist on enforcing strict trade laws aimed at protecting lucrative returns, in the midst of such a disaster, is to say the least insensitive. However, some apologists have come out strongly to contest the widespread demands for an urgent review of these laws, pleading that the situation has been adequately taken care of by the safeguards embedded within TRIPS and patents laws. The professed safeguards include compulsory licensing, parallel importation and a grace period "generously" allowed for the poorest of the poor countries until their "development" caught up. Never mind that AIDS had reversed any developmental achievements in most AIDS devastated countries. Incredibly, a timetable was set by the WTO spelling out when various poor countries had to have passed the necessary laws to make them TRIPS compliant. In the meantime they could in theory import or even manufacture copies of any AIDS drugs without suffering the harsh penalties, provided they followed the correct procedure.

In practice, however, these so-called special considerations to poor countries are almost like a cruel joke. To begin with, the exempted countries by definition are too poor to manufacture the AIDS drugs, especially the very latest, safer and more effective ones, or benefit from other aspects of the "concessionary" laws. Unless such poor countries strike oil and manage it well, there is no chance that they will, within the allotted period or any time soon thereafter, reach the level of development to be fairly harmonised by the same trade laws with the richest countries on earth. This pathetic situation notwithstanding, poor countries were not spared intense pressure to hurry and pass the laws ahead of the grace period. Florid language was used to explain the benefit of enacting such laws early. Kenya was seemingly persuaded into passing the law at a time when there was no necessity or discernible benefit for her to do so, except being promised lucrative trade contracts and open Western markets. Yet soon afterwards, Kenya found that instead of the promised benefits, they had imposed restrictions on themselves including less access to medicines! They have since sought to amend the law.

I found to my dismay that the Ugandan Parliament was on the verge of falling into the same trap as neighbouring Kenya. As usual plenty of funding was made available for the exercise, and the consultants were freely provided to quickly draft the act. Workshops, where generous allowances were paid, were hurriedly arranged and expatriate facilitators flown in to "guide" the discussions. When I heard of what was happening, I put aside my other commitments to blow the whistle on the scheme. I made a presentation to parliamentarians on May, 3 2003, and talked at some of the workshops warning of the grave danger of hurriedly passing foreign, consultants'-led, patents laws. I pleaded that at the very least there was no urgency or obligation to rush the law through, and that it would certainly be counter-productive to do so. A few key people picked up the danger signals and some others started asking questions. The net effect was to slow down the process. However, I am sure that the indomitable consultants and facilitators, who have to justify their hefty fees, did not just close shop. There was too much at stake for that to be allowed to happen. They must have remained busy somewhere in the background trying to figure out other channels to smuggle this law in. The consultants would have been sure that collaborators, who would not ask too many questions, especially when given generous allowances, could always be found in poverty ridden Africa.

The rules and procedures incorporated in "compulsory licensing" are so cumbersome that it ends up being of real benefit mainly to the rich countries, which don't really need the protection. For instance, it is a requirement that any country, which takes up compulsory licensing in order to provide emergency drugs to their people, must first of all notify and justify the need to the patent holder, and then undertake to provide adequate compensation. The difference between payment and compensation is deliberately not precisely defined. It is left to negotiation. If poor countries had such a capacity to negotiate a price, why not just negotiate the purchase of the drugs right away? Under its provision, the law allows the applicant country to manufacture the needed drugs strictly for use in such an emergency within the country and not to sell it to other countries. Just imagine an AIDS-hit poor African country, like Burundi, trying to rush such a law through so as to provide timely life saving HAART to her people. Such a country would have no money to compensate the pharmaceutical companies for their patent. Even if Burundi manufactured the drugs, it would take time to set up the necessary infrastructure while the carnage continued. To go around this, some provisions for importing from more technologically advanced countries would be allowed. However, if such a country offered to help, it would by virtue of being relatively advanced be constrained by the same patents law. A classic Catch-22!

The compulsory licensing law works best if governments take the responsibility for acquiring the licence, though in theory any individual could do it. What if the affected country has a despotic leadership, which refuses to invoke this clause on behalf of her suffering population, or refuses to acknowledge the emergency? However, just in case anyone entertains the thought that this is just a hypothetical question, it actually happened in South Africa. For a long time the leadership refused to endorse life-saving therapy while her citizens died en masse. Shamelessly, even under such sad circumstances, the pharmaceutical companies still went ahead and sued luckless South Africa. There was, no immediate threat to the monopoly of their drugs. There was only mere muttering that the use of low cost generics would be considered by South Africa, without any serious intention to immediately introduce them at the time. The big Pharma cannot have felt threatened by this stance since they were aware that South Africa was at best dragging her feet with regard to the introduction of antiretroviral therapy. Their main concern was fear of setting a precedent. In theory, any individual, charity or humanitarian organisation could have stepped in to take up compulsory licensing if a government was unwilling or unable to act, but they would still need direct, or at least moral, state protection to do it. To underscore the ineffectualness of such a move, if the powerful government was in the dock, then it would just be foolhardy for an individual to dare.

The "grace period" given to some poor countries is just futile. One pharmaceutical company representative once taunted me saying, "Go on make the drugs! What is stopping you? Your country Uganda is not even bound by the patents law yet!" This was precisely the point. The poor countries supposed to benefit from this grace period, purportedly so that they can catch up, could not make any meaningful use of it. It was exactly for this reason that they were granted the grace period in the first place. Countries like India, South Africa and Brazil, which could have benefited from it, were threatened with sanctions and not surprisingly India had to fall in line. The penalty for non-compliance is harsh, because it is meant to be both punitive and a deterrent. It includes trade sanctions and exclusion from the lucrative Western markets. The case of India was particularly worrying because it had been the main country supplying cheap generic drugs to many poor countries. Now they had to conform to the patents law, thus cutting off a vital lifeline for the poor. There was a rush to reassure the poor countries that the law would not affect the current flow of generic AIDS drugs. Such reassurance, however, was just hot air. The low cost drugs being produced by the generic manufacturers include the cheap fixed dose combination formulations of Stavudine, Lamuvudine plus Nevirapine, and Zidovudine, Lamuvudine and Nevirapine marketed by Cipla of India as Triomune, and, Duovir–N respectively. The big Pharma do not feel threatened by Cipla now or other Indian generic drugs manufacturers. Three of the four commonest AIDS drugs they make are no longer in high demand in the West, due to the unacceptably high incidence of side effects and because newer, safer and more effective drugs have become available.

For instance, Stavudine is more commonly associated with a fat metabolic disorder that drains fats out of limbs and faces and deposits it around the abdomen and breasts. Victims' faces are left with a thin layer of skin clinging to the skull and facial bones giving them a wizened appearance that subjects them to stigma. It also causes inflammation of the nerves (peripheral neuropathy) especially in advanced stages of AIDS, which condemns the sufferers to pins and needles and a non-stop burning sensation which in its severe form keeps the affected patients awake for nights on end. In the extreme form, the side effects can be devastating; such as the case of a woman I saw, whose lower limbs were so severely affected that she was brought to my clinic in a wheel chair. With the widespread use of Stavudine in poor countries, following the donor programmes including the global AIDS fund, we witnessed a rising level of life-threatening side effects, including a rise of lactic acid in the blood (lactic acidosis) some of which were fatal. Only in exceptional circumstances is Stavudine used in the West as first line treatment of AIDS. It was taken off the list of first line drugs when safer ones became available. As a result the price plummeted as demand took a nosedive in the West. Guess what? This and other drugs not on demand in the West were the very first ones to be exempted under the new patents law. India may continue to manufacture these generally unwanted and to some extent toxic drugs for poor countries without any problem, but must not make the newer, safer and lucrative drugs on high demand in the West. All the most commercially lucrative AIDS drugs, those relatively free of serious side effects, were introduced after 1996. These are the AIDS drugs of the future. They include Tenofovir, a much safer substitute for the out-of-favour Stavudine or Zidovudine, and Maltrex also marketed as Aluvia a highly effective drug which, unlike the older version Kaletra, does not need to be kept in a fridge - thus more suited to Africa since it is heat stable. Other drugs are in the pipeline. What will happen to the poor patients when all the loopholes for easier access to modern AIDS drugs are blocked as seems to be the plan?

Perhaps the most reprehensible aspect of enforcing the TRIPS and patents law in its present form is that it virtually gives the poor countries a rope to hang themselves with by compelling them to be signatories to these faulty laws. This state of affairs is hard to defend, and future generations will find it mind-boggling that it was found acceptable to a civilised world. This is clear evidence that the strength of the patents lobby is very powerful. For poor countries that regularly suffer lengthy processes to get any kind of international financial assistance, even if it is for a catastrophic emergency like AIDS, consultants to "help" them enact patents laws are freely and readily offered. In fact, such help may not be wantonly refused. That may explain how diverse African countries with totally different legal and political frameworks generally come out with uniform patents laws, looking like it was all achieved voluntarily and independently. The net effect of it all is that the these countries are browbeaten into becoming allies in an exercise that ensures their own doom - with their well-documented consent. In future when this untenable situation is being condemned, as indeed it must, documents will be flashed onto the table to show that it was not the rich countries that turned a blind eye while the "patents weapon of mass destruction" was committing the genocide. A ready alibi is in place well ahead of the supposed tribunal. When the time of judgement comes, the poor countries will with great embarrassment be found holding the smoking gun. The evidence will be self-explanatory. It will show clearly that they voluntarily participated in enacting these laws. Records will evidently show that their own parliaments freely debated and passed them. The little but crucial detail about free consultants who actually drafted the laws will be forgotten or just omitted. No mention will be made of the seminars where members of parliament received generous per diems. Politicians can always be trusted to have debated the issue like it was their very original brilliant idea. People will wonder why rational people decided to pass a law that caused so much anguish and deaths.

There is goodness inherent in humanity. On this platform, it remains the duty of all the people of the world to balance self-centredness perpetuated among us by tiny minority interests, and public and humanitarian interests. As the facts are self evident, it is imperative that all countries get together to correct this situation. Compassion necessitates that legalised injustices should be eliminated from international laws. This will go a long way towards creating a peaceful world. It will help reduce unjustifiable violent acts increasingly being used to address grievances.

Whereas the current so-called TRIPS safeguards are hopeless for poor countries, they work marvellously well for rich countries because they were designed and tailored to their specific needs and means. It is therefore the rich and powerful countries that are almost always the exclusive beneficiaries of the compulsory licensing law. The United States and Canada are the biggest users of compulsory licensing for pharmaceutical products. The United States issued compulsory licences as a means of forcing down drug prices. In the 1960s and 1970s, the US Army produced and used Tetracycline and Meprobamate without authorisation from the patent holders. In 2001, in the face of the threat of bio-terrorism, the US considered issuing a compulsory licence for Ciprofloxacin. In the case of Canada, between 1969 and 1983, it granted an average of twenty compulsory licences per annum for drugs. This practice was a key factor in the development of the mighty Canadian generic drugs industry.

The pharmaceutical companies must be thrilled every time the USA or any other rich G8 country invokes the compulsory licensing law. First of all, it is a clear demonstration that the law works. Secondly, the pharmaceutical companies owe them one. The G8 countries, the eight richest in the world, are their strongest supporters and enforcers of the laws that ensure them high profits. It is a pleasure to have an opportunity to pay back their generous benefactors, especially if they face an emergency like the anthrax threat. The drugs patent holders are further thrilled by the reassurance that under the terms of the compulsory licensing law the rich countries are in a position to pay them a hefty compensation. It is even possible that they will make even more money this way than they would otherwise since a state of emergency is inevitably associated with increased demand. But Canada and USA are not always such good neighbours when it comes to drugs. Canada, with a more liberal public health programme, has lower drugs prices, and some Americans trek across the border for more affordable drugs. This does not find favour with the American-based pharmaceuticals, which are constantly lobbying for punitive action against Canada. However, Canada, unlike many African countries, is no banana republic and caution is the key.

The problem arises only when the poor countries seek to use the same compulsory licensing option for their public health emergencies. They are hit hard by such severe and punitive measures and calculated restrictions that no one else dares to try. Two examples clearly indicate the dilemma. Brazil, a medium-income country, tried to invoke compulsory licensing with a view to developing an industry for generic drugs. Immediately a lobby group of the US pharmaceutical industry started pressurising the office of the US Trade Representative to take retaliatory action. Trade sanctions were threatened, including removal of Brazil from the General Preference System so that it would no longer have duty-free facilities for some of its products in the lucrative US market. Yet humble Brazil was not violating its national or international laws. At the national level, Article 64 of the Industrial Property Law

Number 9.279/96 makes a provision for compulsory licensing on the following grounds: non-utilisation of patents, public interest, national emergency, compensation for non-competitive practices, and in cases where dependent patents exist. At the international level provision is made for compulsory licensing in Article 31 of the Trade Related aspects of Intellectual Property Rights (TRIPS) Agreement of the World Trade Agreement (WTA). Brazil's law guarantees the right to health as defined in Article 196 of the 1988 federal constitution. It is under this law that the country provides free and universal AIDS drugs. Back in the 1980s, the United States started applying Section 301 of their Trade Act, which provides for retaliation against countries adopting trade practices that are contrary to US legal international rights. Brazil was, at the time, one of their targets. Indeed, in 1988, the United States imposed a 100% ad valorem tax on products like paper, chemical and electronics. According to the paper industry, which was one of the most seriously affected, the losses were estimated at US$250 million (Tachmardi, 1993). The imbalances of the current patents laws are quite clear. On June 23, 2005, the editorial of the *New York Times* described Brazil's efforts to guarantee access to ARV treatment under a heading BRAZIL RIGHT TO SAVE LIVES. The editorial suggested among other things that the US Trade Representative should make a public statement that the United States would not retaliate against Brazil for exercising its right to save lives.

South Africa is yet another vivid example. In 2001 the leadership there spoke of introducing generic copies of the AIDS drugs in order to save the lives of their citizens because of mounting pressure and public outcry. Shockingly, 500 South African lives were being lost to AIDS daily, equivalent to a fully loaded Jumbo jet plus a full smaller passenger plane, or fifty fully loaded minibuses crashing and killing everyone on board every day! As explained earlier, at the time the South African government was in denial, openly opposed to AIDS drugs. It was, therefore, on the side of the patents holder by default. Nevertheless, the pharmaceutical companies shamelessly took the AIDS devastated country to court. If Africa's most powerful country, South

Africa, and Brazil, which by most African standards is an enormously rich country, faced serious problems trying to invoke the patents clause, how easy would it be for a miserably poor country to try and acquire compulsory licensing? In practice, therefore, compulsory licensing is just like a cruel hoax on the poor.

However, the lobbyists had a ready strong counter to this query. Unbelievably, Mozambique and Zambia effortlessly surmounted all obstacles that dogged mighty South Africa and Brazil without so much as a drop of sweat and successfully invoked the compulsory licensing law. Amazingly, the impossible seemed to have been pulled off by two of the poorest countries on earth without so much as a hiss or fuss from the highly protective big Pharma. No court cases! It was all smiles and congratulations all round. How did they do it? Patents and TRIPS consultants and lobbyists explain it by saying that it was as easy as cutting a cake. In reality, the countries were allowed to effortlessly succeed in order to demonstrate a token application of the compulsory licensing law by licensing a few AIDS drugs which were already widely available from many other generic manufacturers and no longer in demand in the West. Close scrutiny will clearly show that it had no significant effect with regard to AIDS patients' access to therapy in these countries. It was more useful for propaganda purposes, and a rather cynical vindication of the laws.

No wonder the presumed guardians of the iniquitous law, the G8, are faced with bitter protests whenever they meet. This is because globalisation has rightly or wrongly been linked to socio-economic injustice and human rights. It is in the same context that WTO regulations, TRIPS and patents and their application to life-saving drugs are viewed. Sometimes the G8 puts on their agenda some constructive issues related to the alleviation of the dire situation in poor countries, especially Africa. Sometimes they approve some relief funds. However, such hardly makes any durable impact because they ignore the real cause of the misery, namely poverty and some bad international laws. Otherwise handouts, debt relief and aid are yet another example of mopping the floor while the tap runs.

Julie Davids, the Executive Director of Community HIV/AIDS Mobilisation Project, NYC, said in the film "Pills, Profits And Profits" that "HIV/AIDS is not an unstoppable plague — it is a preventable epidemic and people making a profit and standing in the way of solutions can and must be held accountable." This is yet another voice underscoring the imperative nature of this issue. The current practices must be properly addressed and not merely amended cosmetically. A more humane alternative must be found. It just cannot be true that scientists will stop harnessing science for the well-being of humanity unless humanity pays a heavy price, including the sacrifice of millions of lives. If innovation worked only this way, then it is not the science that we know. It would be like a return to the time of human sacrifices.

Mr Guest saw a solution to all this. He recommends differential pricing whereby the rich countries continue to pay the exorbitant price while the poor African countries pay just a fraction as the answer to this tragedy. Then he goes on to bemoan that when the pharmaceutical companies kindly agreed to this and started providing subsidised AIDS drugs, the incorrigibly corrupt Africans, oblivious to the plight of their fellow suffering Africans, re-exported the drugs back to Europe in order to make a profit. It is indeed true that by the time Mr Guest was writing his book, *The Shackled Continent,* the branded AIDS drugs pharmaceutical companies had made some insignificant reductions and some questionable donations. As described below, some of the so-called reductions, which I personally witnessed, were controversial. Nevertheless, some reductions had become inevitable not necessarily because of the charitable nature of the big Pharma, but as a result of the stiff generic competition. In addition, it was also because some of the drugs fell out of favour in the Western market. As is always the case competition drove the cost down, but it also worked in two directions.

The generic manufacturers, like their counterparts the brand manufacturers, are also unrepentant profiteers despite often posturing to the contrary. As they thrive on drugs mainly not protected by patents law, they respond to the usual market forces, and try to make as much profits as possible. Nevertheless, the net effect of the reductions was that AIDS drugs remained over and above what the vast majority of the people could afford. It was like offering a bare footed village peasant a brand new Rolls Royce at the cost price of a used Mercedes Benz. If it is at all true that anyone re-exported the drugs, as Mr. Guest alleged, then very few if anyone in Africa noticed or suffered as a result. The vast majority of Africans derived no benefit at all from the so-called drugs reductions. The hyped-up symbolic reduction did not make a dent in the desperate situation. For all but a tiny minority the reduction went totally unnoticed. On the contrary, the Africans continued to die in huge numbers. In fact, at that time there was no shortage of the drugs as such; the problem was that they were just not affordable. In such a sad situation, the alleged re-export of the de facto non-existent drugs, as an illustration of the "rampant corruption of Africans", was just unfortunate. Surely there are very many better examples of corruption on the continent like that of Mobutu who built a golden castle for himself. In this context the comparison was at the very worst callous, or at the very best in bad taste. There is an old saying of my tribe that goes: "If you deny help to a drowning man, at least spare him the laughter."

Pharmaceutical companies like all traders are entitled to their share of fair profits, but they must find an ethical way to earn it. They must find a way that does not deny dying poor people a chance to live. Drugs manufacturers need to appreciate that it pays dividends to invest in humanity whether they are poor or not. In the case of AIDS, there are forty million lives at stake, people who need to take the drugs for life. These are excellent potential business partners but only when kept alive. Dead people are not good business partners unless one is either an undertaker or a coffin maker. Happy, healthy people are the basis of successful businesses and a nation's development. They are the peacemakers of the world. That's why almost all commercial adverts depict happy, appreciative and satisfied customers. I refuse to accept that addressing patents and TRIPS would be a nail in the coffin of business. On the contrary, it would be a win-win situation for all. Compassion and human rights never killed initiative or business. They promote it.

A call for fair trade does not denote intellectual piracy, or non-recognition of innovation. It is a call for ethical and humanitarian practices for better trade. However, some other trading practices in the West are far from fair and also need to be addressed. Such unfair trading practices hinder Africa from lifting herself out of the poverty trap. In turn, this results in an inability to tackle catastrophes like AIDS and a dependence syndrome. For instance, agriculture is one of the biggest industries in the West but at least some of the African produce could easily be competitive in the west if there were fair trading practices. This is because of much lower production costs in poor countries and the increased demand for organic produce in the West. But there are strict protectionist laws and red tape that denies access of such products to the lucrative Western markets. Massive subsidies are given out to non-competitive farmers to produce overpriced goods and sometimes to overproduce, blocking any chance of credible competition from poor countries. At one time in Europe they talked of wine lakes and butter mountains. Also, ways have been found to protect jobs from emerging industrial giants, such as China, producing cheaper goods. China, which has recently emerged as an industrial giant, is hitting back with counter threats and measures of her own.

Poverty played a big role in AIDS and continues to do so. Addressing AIDS without addressing poverty is ultimately futile. No powerful country would have tolerated such a massive death toll among its citizens while an effective remedy was denied to them for profit. This could only happen to the weak and marginalised poor peoples of the world. The rich and powerful would have just gone to war as they have often done even for less deserving causes. But in such circumstances it would have been defensible.

Surely there must be a way through which trade and business can work for humanity, while making reasonable profits. There must be a way the world can use advances in science and technology to address humanitarian emergencies and disasters without linking them to devastating profits. There must be other ways to reward scientific breakthrough and innovation. Perhaps as part of the requirements for research to be supported by public funds, it needs to be made mandatory that any commercially exploitable results are made accessible to the public at a fair and affordable price without discrimination against the poor. There must be a straightforward way to empower the resource-constrained countries to access critical drugs without the current charade of unworkable compulsory licensing laws. Although buttons and pills may sometimes look the same, it is just not right to have the same trade laws for both. There must be a way to unleash interventions to save humanity from disease, poverty, natural and other kinds of disasters. As far as mass killer diseases like AIDS are concerned, the current laws have badly let down humanity resulting in untold suffering and millions of preventable deaths. The world must prepare to do better next time.

The Poor Man's AIDS Drug

Until 2003, when some treatment donations started trickling in, the standard of AIDS care and management in Africa was prevention, mild palliatives and the treatment of a few easy-to-treat opportunistic infections. Almost everyone else who needed antiretroviral drugs or expensive therapy for opportunistic infections died. Seminars, workshops and courses specifically targeting resource-constrained countries that addressed only the easy options were funded, and generous per diems were paid out. Only research projects that either tested drugs for opportunistic infections or targeted HIV prevention in Africa were funded. Any applications for funding that involved antiretroviral drugs, like the many good research proposals which the JCRC made, were promptly rejected as neither appropriate nor possible in Africa. Yet this was just blatant hypocrisy that merely added insult to the deaths of the African people. In reality AIDS treatment should have been the number one priority on any research agenda for Africa, as it was the leading killer.

In my case, numerous nasty infections that took advantage of a weakened body known as AIDS Opportunistic Infections (OIs) were so many that they would require a small booklet to list them. The OIs range from minor ailments, usually self limiting in a normal person but turned by AIDS-induced low immunity to severe maiming and life threatening-infections. AIDS also induces some of the most vicious malignant cancers imaginable. The most serious among the diseases include toxoplasmosis, caused by a parasite common in cats' gut. To healthy people it is almost harmless but when it attacks AIDS patients it causes a life-threatening disease. Toxoplasmosis often invades the brain, forming abscesses that cause the sufferers serious convulsions, which go on excruciatingly until they lapse into coma – and until death mercifully ends their misery. Other serious OIs include cytomegalovirus, which slowly dims the vision until the helpless victim becomes completely blind; but, unlike toxoplasmosis, relief in the form of death does not come quickly, thus prolonging the patient's and the family's agony for months. Then there is the dreadful Cryptococcal Meningitis, a fungal infection that swells the brain resulting in an excruciating headache, often described by patients as "bombs exploding in my head". These torturing infections that hit AIDS patients were often not included among the opportunistic infections addressed at the sponsored seminars. Yet they were so common that there was hardly any single day in the 1990s that passed without encountering at least one patient with these horrible diseases. Hospitals across Africa were full of them and other more ghastly AIDS-associated conditions, such as cancers. In all international seminars these killers diseases of Africans were merely glossed over or were conspicuous by their deliberate exclusion. The so-called experts discussed treatment of only a few easy-to-treat OIs, as if these other very serious conditions did not exist.

What were the reasons for the double standards? Did these conditions not have any known therapy? Effective treatment did indeed exist, and this was the good news, but the bad news that zipped the mouths of the so-called experts, humanitarian organisations, WHO and UNAIDS included, was the exorbitant cost of the drugs to treat them. It was indeed cheaper to buy gold than to treat some of these diseases. What was instead being promoted and funded, as the AIDS drug for Africa was a very cheap, widely available antibiotic Cotrimaxazole, widely known in all village shops in most parts of Africa as Septrin or Bactrim. It had no patent protection mainly because much more effective antibiotics were available in the West, and it was therefore being produced unchallenged by virtually all major pharmaceutical plants in almost all poor countries. Because it was widely accessible it had, from the early 1970s, become the poor man's antibiotic of choice after Penicillin and Tetracycline, and was widely used for treatment of everything ranging from sore throats to gonorrhoea. It became one of the most abused drugs and over time many bacterial infections developed resistance to it.

Although it was known to reduce the risk of acquiring some few OIs, it had no effect whatsoever on many other killer AIDS OIs, like cryptococcal meningitis or cytomegalovirus. However, the way it was promoted made it look like an AIDS wonder drug, and some lay people mistakenly even thought it was one of the antiretroviral drugs. In fact, by 2005 Ugandan newspaper editorials were still writing about its "wonder effect." A few studies to define its benefits were carried out and the limited beneficial findings grossly exaggerated, to make Septrin look like a great AIDS drug. In reality, Septrin simply prevented or altered the clinical course of a limited number of opportunistic infections, but certainly did not have any power to stop the deterioration of AIDS patients' immunity. Therefore without antiretroviral therapy, patients would just go on to get one or other of the many other killer opportunistic diseases on which Septrin had no effect. Simply put, treatment of opportunistic infections without concurrent or follow-up ART was just an exercise in futility. Yet this was precisely what was recommended as the poor man's AIDS therapy for Africa. It was partly recommended and selected on the basis of being an easy and very cheap option - a widely available product that did not have patents protection, and therefore was not contentious. In my observations I found that the actual value of Septrin to AIDS patients was quite limited. However, I realise that in such dire circumstances it was better than nothing. In fact, I used Septrin prophylaxis fairly commonly on my patients for all it was worth, as there was just no alternative. But I always explained its limitations.

However, there is at least one condition where Septrin is a wonder drug. The same old cheap, widely available Septrin was found to be a life saver for one very serious opportunistic infection called

Pneumocytis Pneumonia (PCP). PCP attacks the lungs, causing massive inflammation resulting in failure to absorb and exchange oxygen. This is one of the most distressing AIDS opportunistic diseases. Sufferers are some of the most heart-wrenching sights to behold, as they are tortured by a horrifying drowning feeling. Their respiratory rate initially goes up to compensate for the decreasing absorption of oxygen, followed by panting in apparent air hunger, utilising all accessory breathing muscles, intensifying as the drowning feeling worsens. Then panic sets in as the situation deteriorates further. Many victims splash around just like drowning men until exhausted. Mercifully, as the brain gets starved of oxygen, they begin to lose consciousness, followed by gasping even while breathing pure oxygen, until they finally go into coma succumbing to suffocation. Septrin, especially when used early or in combination with steroids, is a lifesaver in this horrific condition. However, because of the serious nature and need for quick and sustained high blood levels, Septrin is best given by intravenous infusion. Many patients in critical need of this life-saving drug died as I watched helplessly, frustrated, and embarrassed. I knew the drug that could have saved their lives yet I could not find any for them. They therefore had to die an agonising but preventable death simply because the intravenous preparation of Septrin was not available.

One widow nursing her daughter with PCP in my ward once attacked me shouting, "There is no oxygen in your pots, doctor. It must be another gas; otherwise my daughter would not be suffocating." She said this in between sobs as she could barely endure to look at the dying daughter. "See - she can't breathe – she has nothing to breathe!" she cried. There was nothing wrong with the oxygen pot, and her mask was well positioned. All she needed was intravenous Septrin to quickly kill the bug in her lungs and reverse the reaction and inflammation that prevented the oxygen entering her blood. Yet all that was available was the oral tablet forms that were crushed and flushed down her tummy through a nasal–stomach tube, but it was just too slow to act through this route.

So what happened to the cheap Septrin produced by almost all poor countries? Why was it not available? The problem was that the killer

PCP was not only a disease of AIDS patients. PCP is also associated with other conditions that cause different forms of immune-suppression including cancer therapy, and immunosuppressive treatment following organ transplants to minimise rejection of alien transplanted organs and tissues. The intravenous formulation of Septrin was therefore in very high demand in the rich Western countries where these conditions were common. In this form, Septrin minted money for the pharmaceutical companies that made it specifically for the lucrative Western market. Therefore, to protect profits, the technology for its manufacture was not readily transferred to Africa. As the poor countries did not manufacture it, it remained unaffordable to the poor Africans. It was obviously not too expensive because of "the need to recoup research and development funds" (the usual excuse) since the patent protection had long expired and whatever was used to develop it long recovered, but it was yet another clear example of profits above lives.

AIDS papers published in the 1980s and early 1990s used to state that PCP was rare in Africans with AIDS. This was false. It was a difficult disease to make an evidence-based diagnosis, and it could be easily confused with many other respiratory opportunistic infections, especially tuberculosis and pneumonia. Yet it was there all the time torturing and killing patients. True, the cheap Septrin tablets used prophylactically could reduce the chances of getting this dreadful PCP, but many patients presented themselves for the first time to health facilities with established PCP required life saving intravenous preparation. Even those who used Septrin for prevention, without ART, would still die from some other opportunistic infections, some of them just as excruciating, on which Septrin had no effect. Therefore whenever I got the opportunity to be present at seminars that discussed "the wonders of Septrin", I would always emphasize the urgent need for ART in addition to the prophylaxis. I would reject the claims that the poor could not use ART, which was then the usual excuse. Such insensitive misinformation used to upset me and still does.

While Septrin was being promoted as the poor man's AIDS drug, problems associated with the use of ART in poor countries were grossly exaggerated, so as to appear insurmountable. Some people, who perhaps knew better, but still threw scares about ART use in poor countries, appalled me. This lie was repeated so often that many believed it. Incredibly some still believe it today.

UNAIDS ART drugs Access Initiative

Back in 1997, the AIDS drugs manufacturers continued to resist any drugs cost reduction despite a worldwide outcry and sustained activist pressure. Yet, naturally, they wanted to maintain a good corporate image. Besides the pharmaceutical companies, WHO and UNAIDS were also on the spot and feeling the heat. UNAIDS then regularly posted new and increasingly gloomy AIDS statistics like cricket scores, without the corresponding action to curtail the epidemic. It was, therefore, facing widespread criticism for its failure to respond to the plight of the poor being decimated by AIDS, though in all fairness it was difficult to see what they could have done when the rich countries that normally provide them with funding support were standing looking on. As some sort of world health brokers charged with the alleviation of AIDS, the beleaguered UNAIDS had a common interest with the pharmaceutical companies, though for dissimilar reasons, in starting a dialogue about the price of drugs.

As the discussions got underway, I witnessed some astonishing twists and turns by pharmaceutical companies in an effort to protect their business monopoly and profits cleverly camouflaged as great, compassionate, humanitarian donations. In one such manoeuvre, some pharmaceutical companies formed what appeared to me an unworkable consortium, ostensibly to provide reduced cost ARV drugs to poor African patients. It was an amazing stage-managed scheme designed to look like the big Pharma would drastically cut the cost of their drugs. It was complete with a fall-back position to address issues raised by anyone who could see through the smokescreen. Whenever we asked when our poor patients back in Africa could expect to see delivery of affordable drugs, a ready explanation was that the mechanism to achieve it was already in place and all that was required was to have patience and give it time to work. Yet to all practical intents and purposes, it started looking more and more like a public relations exercise.

At the time it was quite apparent that no pharmaceutical company was prepared to consider the reduction of the cost of their drugs. In fact, I got an impression that no company could do so even if it had the will, without being in breach of the so-called "fair trade" understanding, and solidarity within the drugs industry. Also, there were fears within the industry that reductions could trigger similar demand from the money-spinning Western consumers, thus jeopardising profits. Therefore, no drugs company could dare break ranks. Yet pressure, mainly from activists and humanitarian international organisations, including the Nobel Prize winning MSF, for cost reduction was mounting by the day.

From November 1996 to June 1997, a number of meetings were held in Geneva, involving government officials from developing countries, NGOs and some people living with AIDS. They discussed possible interventions to increase AIDS drugs access. Starting from June 1997, more follow-on meetings were arranged by UNAIDS in Geneva, involving the AIDS drugs pharmaceutical companies, patents experts, AXIOS (a private company based in Ireland that seemed to play a middleman's role), and some token delegates from the affected "resource constrained" countries. I presume I was one of the token delegates though I personally attended as a horror-stricken doctor looking for something - anything - that would be of some relief to my suffering patients. I arrived in Geneva with guarded optimism that something would be done for my suffering patients. I was armed with all the information about the horrors of AIDS that surrounded me on daily basis and hoped that this would galvanise the big Pharma and UNAIDS to scramble some relief. The meeting however, was not interested in those details. In fact UNAIDS knew it all. The agenda had only one topic for consideration. It was negotiation of an accord under which the drugs companies could provide lower cost ARV drugs to poor countries while protecting their monopoly and prices.

As a novice in such meetings involving interests of big businesses, I was taken aback by the conditions set by the big Pharma for attendance. First of all, they insisted on a cast-iron confidentiality pact and required that all participants sign a document committing them to silence.

Some of the pharmaceutical companies agreed to participate only in the presence of their lawyers. In other words, they had agreed to the meeting with the express aim of protecting their lucrative business interests, and were not prioritising cost reductions or at least making any meaningful concession. It was a bad omen. In one of the meetings where I was involved I witnessed some of the big Pharma lawyers openly restrain their clients from making any statements or any promises that could in any way be construed as a kind of compromise or commitment on their part to lowering the cost of their drugs. I could feel my heart begging: "Please, please have mercy."

As far as I could discern, these meetings were just an exercise in futility. However, on the side of UNAIDS and the big Pharma, both anxious for positive publicity, it achieved some important objectives by the mere fact that the meetings actually took place and that delegates from AIDS-devastated poor countries participated. This was portrayed as a transparent exercise involving the poor countries concerned - the intended beneficiaries - fully participating in the crucial decision making process and sharing in the successes and failures. There was also an additional advantage in involving the poor countries, and perhaps the most important one was that they would share the blame if it all flopped, which looked like the most likely outcome.

Meanwhile back in Africa, the AIDS-plagued poor countries were hopeful that something serious was being done about the prices. Their hope was raised to expect that help would soon be on the way and the press releases from Geneva did not report otherwise. The sworn silence of participants would ensure they remained with their misconception, while the big Pharma carried on with their business as usual.

Eventually on June, 16 1996, in yet another crisis meeting that included executives of pharmaceutical companies, a deal was struck with UNAIDS to support the establishment of an amazingly designed pilot phase. However, to seal this deal the big Pharma set more conditions aimed at entrenching their monopoly interests. They insisted that any government participating in the pilot scheme must agree to provide protection of intellectual rights of drugs purchased through the initiative, even if they were under no obligation by the TRIPS agreement to do so. This meant that they would offer free police protection of their products from competitors, especially lower cost generics. In return, the only "concession" which the big Pharma made was to undertake to register their products with the National Drugs Authorities in the pilot countries. In fact, this was a routine requirement for registration of any pharmaceutical products in virtually all countries. When this agreement was secured, the reassured big Pharma made an offer, which poor countries could not refuse, as they were desperate for any kind of help. They offered to support a pilot phase in four developing countries identified by UNAIDS, namely Uganda, Cote d'Ivoire, Vietnam and Chile. The choice was partly based on geographical considerations and equity considerations. The big Pharma agreed to channel their support only through clearing houses dubbed "The Non-profit Companies" expressly set up and owned by the pharmaceutical companies themselves in each participating country. The idea was that if it worked well, then the prototype would be duplicated everywhere. The real purpose of this exceptional pilot phase was dubious even at its very best. Was it, for instance, aimed at finding out whether genuine and meaningful cost reductions would be acceptable? Anyhow, the UNAIDS' bandwagon at long last had something to sing about.

Following the landmark deal, a special press conference was called in November 1997 in Geneva to announce, *"UNAIDS ART drugs Access Initiative"*. The accompanying press release optimistically talked about the interest on the part of pharmaceutical companies "to make drugs more affordable," though in reality no such commitment or serious interest existed. However, the silver lining was the concession by the big Pharma that their drugs were not affordable. Next, the release talked about the "role of national governments to improve health infrastructure", without mentioning the definition of a sufficiently improved infrastructure satisfactory to the big Pharma in order to unleash their drugs. Not that they needed to spell it out, since infrastructure was as usual just a red herring, and the hackneyed justification for denial of ART to AIDS sufferers in Africa. The stage was all set for a depressing circus. Only three pharmaceutical companies agreed to join this fundamentally flawed initiative. Others, of course, had better things to do.

Basically the so-called *Non-Profit Companies (NPC)* were planned to work in an ingenious way. However, a warning is called for at this stage, as the reader may be tempted to laugh it off as a bad joke, whereas it actually happened! ...The arrangements were such that the pharmaceutical companies would purchase their own drugs from their own factories in Europe or USA at the international price and export the same drugs to *themselves* through their own NPCs! Confused? Not to worry because this was all according to plan. Anyone curious enough to check the prices would have found that the drugs were being bought and exported at the same cost as in Western countries. No unfair trade. The big Pharma solidarity caucus would be reaffirmed. So the million-dollar question was: Where were the desperately needed reductions supposed to come from? You can bet that the ever-resourceful big Pharma had it all figured out. And it was so simple. The pharmaceutical companies were to use their strong lobby to raise funds for their very own NPCs, which would then subsidise the drugs cost to the consumers, the poor Africans. A win-win situation: the pharmaceutical companies would maintain their prices while the poor Africans would get their much craved for reductions. The representatives of the big Pharma talked in vivid terms of their grandiose plans to sell the scheme to generous rich old widows in Europe and the USA, so that they could make generous wills leaving their superfluous wealth to the clearing houses. To top it up, they proposed that their companies would donate any drugs they could not sell in the West like those about to expire, or sell at a "give away" price any drugs that no one in the rich countries needed, such as those returned by patients to pharmacies. They also planned to lobby humanitarian agencies and foundations for donations. This way, they hoped to raise sufficient funds to provide cheaper drugs without cutting costs and profits, or setting a precedent that would spell doom for the future of their lucrative empire. Above all, they had it all planned to be accomplished without investing so much as a penny of their own money.

Not surprisingly, the scheme flopped miserably. Charitable old ladies just did not die, or at least not in sufficient numbers to leave the kind of money that would make any difference to the cost. No significant donations materialised from other sources either. This was indeed a predictable situation because most donors considered AIDS therapy for the huge numbers of poor victims in Africa a no-go area, courtesy of the propaganda machine that projected problems associated with the provision of ART in Africa as insurmountable. The huge demand for drugs and the colossal amount of money that would be required was usually referred to as "a bottomless pit." Most importantly, no sane donor would make any donations to the pharmaceutical companies which were many times richer than almost all non-governmental donors in the world put together. On the contrary, instead of the promised cost reduction, the cost of drugs actually shot up simply because the clearing houses needed to charge overheads in order to pay local staff, including the boards that were established in each of the participating countries to go through the motions of overseeing the ill-fated venture. Shamefully, the big Pharma were not even ready to fund this very basic need, which would have been a priority if they really had any faith in the success of their own programme. Meanwhile, the promise of the reduced cost of drugs subdued the rising humanitarian activist pressure for at least a little while as business continued as usual.

The outcome of the project was a foregone conclusion, as it was a stillbirth. It did not even take off in Vietnam, because that socialist country saw nothing in it but profiteering and gave it the cold shoulder. Chile, on the other hand, really did not need the initiative for two simple reasons. First of all, it had only a small number of AIDS patients; and secondly, the country was rich enough to treat them all without the gimmicks of the initiative. Cote d'Ivoire abandoned it half way when it realised that there were no discernible benefits. Only Uganda plodded on with little to show for it, except the NPC, or the Clearing House as it was variously called, that survived to a great extent on the Joint Clinical Research Centre's own treatment programme, which had been set up independently long before this initiative.

Eventually even the NPC in Uganda shook off any humanitarian pretence and transformed into an overt profit-making company. Eventually, but perhaps not surprisingly, it was taken over by the very same company that had acted as the middleman in earlier UNAIDS meetings in Geneva. However, the initiative's propaganda bandwagon was so successful in sowing disinformation that some people actually believed it achieved something. Sadly, the worldwide misconception about the initiative was used ruthlessly and caused misery to many AIDS patients. These included a number of them who were deported from the UK (as recounted earlier) on the pretext that they would access free treatment under this flawed initiative that had started with so much promise, but ended as a disappointing circus.

Accelerated Access Initiative

By May 2000, the Pharmaceutical companies and UNAIDS were back again on stage for the second round following the first act that failed to produce any price reductions or significant increase in the numbers of Africans accessing antiretroviral drugs. The big Pharma were forced back by a rapidly rising outcry and resurgence of activist pressure. They could see that the generic drugs manufacturers were rapidly catching up with their cheaper but quality copies of some of the AIDS drugs. Worse still, the generic drugs manufacturers' own promotion campaigns had successfully publicised them as a credible alternative source of AIDS drugs, moreover, at an affordable price. To the poor countries in desperate need of drugs the generic manufacturers increasingly looked like compassionate saviours at the expense of the big Pharma whose drugs were then only for the rich. Therefore, the new programme had to come under a different cover - a sort of air freshener to smother the stench of the failed first initiative.

The new initiative was planned to achieve drugs cost reduction through dialogue as opposed to the first one that was supposed to achieve it through a "smart" business scheme. The strategy seems to have been that as long as the dialogue was in progress the activist pressure would ease; the generics threat would be kept at bay; and the business would not be under so much pressure. The United Nations

(UN), WHO, and especially UNAIDS, also facing unprecedented criticism and pressure, were seriously concerned about the escalating AIDS crisis and were frantically trying to find a solution. Failure to find help for the poor victims of the AIDS scourge was glaringly embarrassing as a sore on the world's human rights face. It was, therefore, time for a corporate image polish up, and intervention on the WHO and UNAIDS side too, especially as they shared blame for the first botched initiative. This time, the participation of the pharmaceutical companies was bigger. Five multinationals got together with UNAIDS and held another round of what was described as "successful talks" which ended with another "historic" agreement by the pharmaceutical companies to "drastically" lower the cost of their products, in order to increase access. The seriousness of this meeting was underscored by the participation of UN in the negotiations. However, the generic drugs manufacturers were not invited to the party in Geneva. I presume that it was considered imperative that the brand manufacturers - the patent holders - were not to be upset. Yet Cipla of India offered one of the best deals, as it could sell generic formulations of the same drugs at almost a third of the price. Evidently, the generic competition must have been an important factor in making the cost reduction offer.

The new programme was baptised rather ironically "Accelerated Access Initiative (AAI)", a very strange choice of name considering that it was coming right on the heels of the botched "UNAIDS Access Initiative!" This time, however, UNAIDS was dropped from the programme title. Who wants to associate his name with a doomed agenda? Almost a year after the initiative I was not surprised that there was still nothing to show. Meanwhile, our expectant patients, whose hope had been raised once more, continuously asked when they would see the reduction.

Meanwhile, at the UN the apparently frustrated Secretary General, Kofi Annan, had expected that the pharmaceutical companies would somehow come to his rescue because he was also under pressure at a global level to do something about the crisis. He convened an emergency meeting in Amsterdam with the pharmaceutical companies, which took place in April 2001. Once again the pharmaceutical companies, including Boehringer Ingelheim, Bristol-Myers Squibb, GlaxoSmithKline, Hoffman-LaRoche and Merck, pledged their support to the treatment access programme. The meeting was as usual hailed as a success and again the pharmaceutical companies agreed "to continue to accelerate the price reduction of HIV/AIDS medicines, particularly for the least developed countries in Africa." After the meeting Secretary General Annan sounded upbeat. "The epidemic is the greatest public health challenge of our times and we must harness the expertise of all sectors of society. The pharmaceutical industry is playing a crucial role" he said. On my side I could see no basis for such excitement about this development if it could be so called. By this time I had a good idea of the egocentric interests of the pharmaceutical industry and their determination to stick to their returns.

Perhaps in an effort to show that the initiative was producing some results, in November 2001 AAI had some news. However, the news, as I expected, was disheartening. They reported that 27,000 people, even then widely believed to be a highly exaggerated figure, in countries *supported* through Accelerating Access initiative were on ART. Considering that millions needed therapy, AAI would have been better advised to keep quiet, if it had not been so desperate for news - any news - to report. The numbers were far too low for the simple reason that the drugs' price remained unaffordable, as there had been no meaningful cost reduction. By the second year of the initiative, the situation was unchanged and on May, 15,2002, it was in many aspects worse. Some frustrated activists described AAI as a "puppet of the pharmaceutical industry." The activists accused the pharmaceutical companies of setting up the partnership with UNAIDS only to help them cling on to their monopoly and harness maximum profits while avoiding egg on their face. The initiative also kept the generic competitors away from the centre of world health policy and funds. At the time the WHO had estimated that about 10 million people, most of them in Africa, were in dire need of immediate antiretroviral therapy, yet the AAI estimated that they were reaching only 0.1% of this number! That this fruitless programme was getting so much publicity for almost no result at all troubled me.

Many humanitarian organisations, including Oxfam International, Doctors Without Borders (Médecins Sans Frontières) and my own Joint Clinical Research Centre, greatly criticised AAI for not including generic drug manufacturers in the initiative. I was one of those leading the campaign for affordable drugs for Uganda and Africa in general so that we could save some lives of our people. The injustice was glaringly clear. The reason why the vast majority of our patients were suffering and dying was simply that they could not afford the life-saving AIDS drugs. It was apparent that the brand pharmaceutical companies were unwilling to make any meaningful reduction on their drugs. Therefore, there being no other sources of help, I continued working on my own trying to find an alternative. In so doing, as described later, I was to discover that this was practically the same as taking on the world.

One activist group in their statement of July, 19, 2002, described Accelerating Access Initiative as "a striking example of a dishonest compromise between international institutions and the pharmaceutical industry at the expense of people and public health." Some people may hear this and wonder whether it was the usual activist rhetoric ,but in my case I saw the futility of this partnership in action. It flopped miserably. Painfully, I saw with my own eyes so many people die who could have lived, while waiting for the promised drugs that were never meant to be. This was cruel.

Meanwhile, the offer by Cipla to provide lower cost AIDS drugs so excited many of us, including Dr Bernard Pecoul, director of the Access to the Essential Medicines Project for Doctors Without Borders(MSF). Dr Pecoul began to see a wider use of ART in their programmes. He said at the time, "This will let us start up our pilot projects on a larger scale." I had come to the same conclusion much earlier and had already taken steps to find ways and means of making the lower cost drugs available at the JCRC in Uganda. At that time, the scaling up of ARVs in poor countries was faced with propaganda, which cited the need for intensive laboratory monitoring of patients on ART, saying that this was impossible in Africa. Instead, some of these so-called experts, who to me appeared more like sadists, suggested that all that could be done for Africa was the provision of clean water, treatment of malaria and the provision of condoms. Interestingly in hindsight, at the time nobody advocated abstinence from sex as the only effective AIDS preventive strategy. This was to come much later and caused so much controversy when substantial prevention funding materialised.

With regard to the propaganda about the crucial need for laboratory monitoring as a basis for denial of therapy to poor countries, the Doctors Without Borders and my centre always insisted that the Western testing standards were over cautious because they could be afforded and their state of epidemic was not in a crisis stage. In our experience using ARVs at the JCRC, we never found any difficulty other than most of our patients' failure to afford the exorbitant cost of the drugs. In any case in a crisis like AIDS, imperfect treatment was better than none at all. The essential test was, of course, HIV testing, and clinical follow-up alone in our dire circumstances would have been enough to start the therapy as long as adherence was good. Adherence did not require or depend on a barrage of sophisticated laboratory testing. Yet it is the major determinant of treatment outcome.

As long as poor conditions in resource constrained countries were accepted as an excuse to deny life saving AIDS drugs, the pharmaceutical companies had a safe alibi. Asked to comment, one pharmaceutical executive characteristically said, "We offer a standard quality from the original manufacturer and can meet any demand that exists out there that can be delivered with safe procedures." The emphasis on "safe procedures" was deliberately used to explain away the horror of AIDS in Africa and elsewhere as just unfortunate and inevitable. As usual the implication was that it was not the exorbitant cost of the drugs to blame but the infrastructure constraints in Africa. As part of the offer to cut the price the same official was challenged further to name the price at which his company would provide the drugs but tactfully refused to do so. Instead he dismissively responded with yet another evasive excuse, "Affordability is an issue, but not the major issue." It was back to the red herring again! Yet we in poor countries who witnessed the daily anguish of AIDS patients had absolutely no doubt that the exorbitant price was the main constraint to ART access, and therefore contributed a lot towards the mammoth numbers of deaths.

However, in a not unexpected turn-around, the usually tight-lipped pharmaceutical company spokesman was to transform into a megaphone as he announced a "generous" offer of free Nevirapine to prevent HIV transmission from mother to child in poor countries. Very generous indeed, until you read the small print - which unfortunately most countries failed to do.

Needless to say, at the end of it all, the Accelerated Access Initiative achieved nothing substantial. Africa remained stuck in her appalling situation that was deteriorating by the day. AIDS deaths in 2002 reached a new high. Hardly anyone noticed the effect of this flawed initiative for the simple reason that there was almost none. However, when you consider that the aim was merely dialogue, someone somewhere will come forward and claim some success, since no one can tell what comes out of any dialogue; especially as the initiative had not set any goals to achieve.

Saving the Little Ones.

As the new millennium got underway, the AIDS bloodbath in Sub-Saharan Africa was relentlessly on the rise. AIDS treatment remained inaccessible as incessant humanitarian appeals for affordable antiretroviral drugs to stop the carnage were ignored. Meanwhile, the donors refused to fund the cost of treatment for the poor, also citing unaffordable prices of the drugs. In various cities all over the world big protest rallies were organised by activists and human rights organisations, and more were planned building up to a massive protest match scheduled to take place at the big International AIDS conference due to take place in Durban, South Africa - the world's most AIDS battered country. As the Durban AIDS conference approached, activists made it abundantly clear that they would vigorously protest against the big Pharma's continued excessive "profiteering" while millions of poor people continued to die a preventable death. Although protests had become part and parcel of every AIDS conference, this particular one was special. The host, South Africa, alone had almost as many people infected with HIV as the entire populations of neighbouring Lesotho, Swaziland and Botswana combined. Without ART all of these people would be destined to die within a decade or so, mostly in their prime and most productive age. Yet many more were still being infected daily. In the southern African region in general, the situation was horrendous. For instance, in neighbouring Lesotho, one in five adults was HIV positive, and the hospital corridors in the mountain kingdom were full of dying AIDS patients seeking non-existent treatment. The overwhelmed and grossly understaffed doctors attended only to the very sick leaving the others to be seen by the dwindling nursing staff. The other nurses, lucky to survive AIDS, had left for greener pastures in South Africa or Europe while their desperately needed services were deputised to nursing aids. On the other side of the South African border, in Botswana, one of Africa's richest countries, the life expectancy had nose-dived to a miserable thirty-seven years because of AIDS. Meanwhile, HIV infected mothers continued to pass on the disease to their babies when effective medicine existed but was out of reach because of the price. The future for Sub-Saharan Africa in general looked bleak. It was an ugly scenario. Yet this tragedy was still happening after one of the greatest scientific breakthroughs of all times - the discovery of antiretroviral drugs (ART) that could have reversed or at least improved the situation. ART had the potential to avert the massacre, and, in the case of Nevirapine, to save hundreds of thousands of babies from HIV/AIDS.

These lucrative drugs became the most protected in history by the patents laws that practically denied life to millions. Understandably, all the international AIDS conferences meant to discuss the scientific progress against AIDS became major occasions for protests against this glaring inequity. What indeed was the use of bringing together so many professionals and civil society representatives from AIDS-devastated countries, presenting to them clear scientific breakthroughs and advances in AIDS treatment that could save their people, and at the end of it all send them home to watch helplessly as their people died? The corporate image of the pharmaceutical companies continuing their business as usual under such dire circumstances had reached "a new level of stench", as some activists put it. It was time again for some air freshener.

At the Durban conference, Boehringer Ingelheim (BI) was targeted for protest among others, but this time round there was an added sense of urgency which the pharmaceutical companies feared most. The increasing demand for the licensing of cheaper generic copies of life-saving AIDS drugs was gathering pace. This threat touched on their central nervous system – profits. Therefore, the stage was set for a clash. Indeed, the conference opened with a big protest march through the streets of Durban, and the big Pharma's stalls were besieged even before they could officially open.

Then out of the clear blue skies one of the pharmaceutical companies, Boehringer Ingelheim, seemingly broke ranks and came up with a solo donation of their product Nevirapine, marketed under the trade name Viramune. Perhaps it was the need to improve their corporate image, but, to be positive, let us assume that it was their spirit of charity that was behind the surprise announcement made in Durban, South Africa, on July, 7 2000. Whatever the reasons the sudden offer caused a stir of excitement in AIDS-devastated countries and took most AIDS activists by surprise. "At long last!" was the common expression of relief by many AIDS patients who came to know about it, rejoicing that their prayers had finally been answered. However, the excitement was short lived.

I was right there in Durban attending the conference, when I heard of BI's announcement to offer free Nevirapine to some African countries, including Uganda. But I did not join in the fanfare because I thought it was just too good to be true. I had been disappointed repeatedly, and therefore I was many times shy. I very well knew that the big Pharma aimed to protect their lucrative business, which was natural for a trading company. The problem, however, was the fact that they had a monopoly of powerful drugs that determined whether an AIDS patient lived or died. The pharmaceutical status quo resulted in all poor patients failing to access the drugs. The memory of the big Pharma's previous offers, including the so-called "UNAIDS HIV Drug Access Initiative" and "Accelerated Access Initiative", were still vivid in my mind. I continued to see signs that the big Pharma, despite their efforts to polish up their corporate image, were digging in their heels to resist the mounting pressure to make any meaningful concession on the cost of their products. At every turn they aimed at fighting off the new threat from generic spoilers. The flurries of announcements that never seemed to produce results could have been just valves for letting off the steam of the activists who were a continued embarrassment to them. I therefore did not think that there was any substantial change. I remained staunchly indifferent to the offer by BI until I met their representative face to face in the boardroom of the Ugandan Ministry of Health. He was giving a presentation on the terms and conditions of their specific free Nevirapine offer to Uganda. The details, though quite predictable, still dismayed me.

The background to the Nevirapine donation goes back to the time in the late 1990s when it was shown in a groundbreaking study conducted in Uganda that it reduced HIV infection from mother to child. It was a breakthrough that offered the very first effective and affordable treatment capable of significantly reducing the deaths from AIDS among babies born to HIV-infected mothers in poor countries. The sheer simplicity of the treatment meant that it could save hundreds of thousand of babies. It did not involve complicated dosaging or laboratory tests. The treatment simply consisted of just one tablet of Nevirapine given to an HIV infected pregnant woman at the onset of labour and a few drops of the syrup of the same drug given to her new born baby. The drug did not require special storage or distribution conditions, and involved small volumes making it easy to use anywhere and at any time. The added advantage was that it did not need any special infrastructure; and, therefore, appeared ideally suited for immediate use in virtually all poor settings.

At the time of the July 2000 announcement, BI's monopoly production of Nevirapine was facing a severe challenge and competition as generic drugs manufacturers had started making copies of it at only a small fraction of the BI price. It is not clear whether the generic challenge was a factor in BI's decision, but it appears that the background to the surprise announcement was much more complex than that. However, as described later, it was to become highly controversial.

Although Nevirapine was being celebrated as a groundbreaking treatment in poor countries, its use as a single drug (monotherapy) for prevention of HIV transmission from mother to child was totally unacceptable in USA or Europe. There, it would have caused a deafening uproar of protests, because it was far below the established standard of care. The standard therapy in the West was a highly efficacious but expensive combination of drugs, which had very impressive outcome far beyond that achievable with Nevirapine alone. Therefore, in comparison, BI's donation to Africa was not only inferior but would be considered grossly unethical in the West. For the poor countries on the other hand, despite the glaring shortcomings, use of Nevirapine in the absence of any other accessible alternative therapy would be considered ethical and acceptable because of the humanitarian need to reduce the high death toll of the little babies. It was also ultimately sustainable in resource constrained countries considering that a dose for the mother consisted of only one pill, which made it cheap when compared to the Western standard treatment. Perhaps this was one of the considerations taken into account when BI made the generous free offer. However, the reason why it was so cheap was not merely that it involved a small dose but also because the demand in the lucrative Western market was declining.

The Durban announcement was particularly significant in what it did not say. For instance, it omitted the disturbing detail that the offer was strictly for only one tablet and a few drops of the syrup each to the poor HIV-infected pregnant women and their new born babies respectively. This was irrespective of whether the mothers needed AIDS treatment for their own lives or not. Absolutely nothing else! There was to be no life-saving antiretroviral therapy for the mother, her baby or family if they were found to need it. The net effect of this donation was that the rescued child would be condemned to the uncertain life of an orphan if the mother who needed treatment was not treated. Such children would have much reduced chances of surviving childhood transmissible infections. There was absolutely no other help offered to the mothers, not even a sponsored information programme aimed at educating them about safer infant feeding. This meant that many babies initially protected from perinatally transmitted HIV would still get it from breast milk as many poor mothers could neither afford formula milk nor be able to prepare it safely.

Almost immediately after the surprise announcement, the Boehringer Ingelheim bandwagon hit the highway to explain the donation to the beneficiaries. At the helm was Ryad Mahfouz, a senior official of BI. A beautiful picture of him was taken as he posed handing over two small packages of Nevirapine to Dr Léon-Alfred Opimbat, Health Minister of the Republic of Congo, on October 20, 2000. Putting aside his usual suit, the honourable minister donned a doctor's clinical white coat, for the picture. However, the picture did not show any big containers full of Viramune in the background for the simple reason that there were none. To be sure, if there had been any such consignment, it would have been too good a photo opportunity to miss. In fact, there was no such consignment on board any ship to deliver the emergency supplies to Congo or any other beneficiary country for that matter. In reality, the size of the small packages without the fancy wrappings was about right to fully accommodate the entire amount of usable Nevirapine tablets for Congo for an entire year. Also posing, for another publicity shot were some medical personnel at Talanghaï Hospital, a childbirth unit in Brazzaville. The pictures were posted with others on the BI website to mark and publicise the generous donation. This was followed by a BI publication on November 28, 2000, entitled "World AIDS Day Report: First supplies in the VIRAMUNE® donation programme for developing countries," to further advertise the donation.

"We believe providing VIRAMUNE® to HIV-positive pregnant women in our country will significantly reduce the number of new infections we see every year in the Congo," the excited Health Minister of the Republic of Congo was quoted in the BI report. Evidently to poor Congo and indeed many poor African countries the Nevirapine donation was the best news ever for their Ministry of Health as far as AIDS treatment was concerned. BI, too, was over the moon, and understandably in expansive mood. Their donation agenda was proceeding very smoothly and getting good applause. "Studies have demonstrated that VIRAMUNE® can fill a critical need in the developing world," Rolf Krebs, Vice-Chairman of the board of managing directors at Boehringer Ingelheim, elaborated. "We're confident that our initiative will continue to increase access to this important drug and will have a considerable impact in the developing world," he elaborated.

However, BI's donation, instead of exciting the activists, provoked their wrath. They described it on the day following the announcement as "amorphous and spurious!" With regard to the confidence expressed by BI that the donation would have considerable impact in the developing world, nothing of the sort actually happened. However, many were misled into thinking that the problem of mother to child HIV transmission had been adequately addressed in poor countries. On the contrary, the project, like all previous ones, began to die off as activist pressure eased, and as the press lost interest and switched to other more newsworthy items. Meanwhile, little babies continued to get AIDS and die, as the highly publicised BI rescue initiative flopped.

Three years later on August 5, 2003, with hardly anything significant to show for the first round of their "donation" programme, BI was back on stage to announce yet another donation. It turned out to be just an extension of the first one, purportedly making it much bigger by opening it up to more countries. Of course, there was no mention of the specific impact of their first phase donation among participating countries. BI simply announced that forty-four countries in Africa, Eastern Europe, Asia and the Caribbean were already benefiting from their free Nevirapine donation. In reality the majority of the people in those target countries did not even know that there was such a programme. "The donation is available to any government expressing interest in national care programmes," as if there was any that didn't, "but also to non-governmental organisations, charitable organisations or other healthcare providers with comprehensive programmes for prevention of Mother-to-Child Transmission," the announcement spelt out.

Yet there was no poor country with such a "comprehensive" programme. The exorbitant cost of the drugs never allowed it to happen. If there had been any country with a "comprehensive programme for prevention of Mother-to-Child Transmission" then by definition it would not have needed the donation. Still, this was no mere careless rhetoric. The words were selected very carefully, and meant exactly what they stated. In time, once again, they would come in handy to explain the inevitable outcome of the donation.

The enticing part of the BI donation announcement was the offer of 166,365 doses of the life-saving drug Nevirapine. I found this style of announcing a drugs donation very interesting. It was one of the rare occasions when a drugs donation was publicised in doses, without a corresponding announcement of its cost in US dollars or some other interchangeable currency. I wondered whether this was an oversight on the part of BI. The figure in doses strangely enough exceeded the figure of the cost in US dollars.

Meanwhile, the BI board chairman, Rolf Krebs, had doors opened for him in high places in AIDS-battered poor countries as he travelled around to explain the donation. The mere mention of doses of a life-saving drug running into hundreds of thousands must have been enough reason to roll out a red carpet for him. BI's statement mentioned that their leader got easy access to government heads and personally led the drive to publicise the donation. His mission, the statement elaborated, "involved talking to governments about the benefits of the donation and the need for expansion of the national healthcare system" among other things. I presume this was needed to accommodate the 'massive' drugs donation, which his company was anxious to deliver, but was somehow constrained by inaction on the part of governments. Nobody raised an eyebrow, as the legendary inefficiency and corruption endemic in Africa was well known.

"We need faster establishment of health infrastructure such as laboratories, trained health personnel, pharmacies and hospitals," Rolf Krebs bemoaned in his statement in order to bring attention to the "frustrating infrastructure constraints." But the offer to help in the rectification of these crucial constraints was not part of the package. Nevertheless, there was a sigh of relief in Africa as the news spread of the very first apparently huge donation - enough to save hundreds of thousands of poor children from being born with the killer disease. In turn, African governments, thirsty for any good news since the AIDS outbreak, capitalised on the unprecedented generous pronouncement and publicised the great news to their AIDS tormented populations. The donation was read out over and over again on radios, and covered widely on both local and international TV channels. The print media flashed the donation as a headline story.

At first glance, the figure of 166,365 doses being donated looked like BI was seriously making an extremely big-hearted donation aimed at saving a vast number of poor children in poor countries. This was the impression until one glanced at the World Health Organisation announcement released at about the same time that put the figures at over 800,000 new infections from mother to child annually. This meant that the numbers of mothers who needed to use Nevirapine was at least two to three times higher annually, and for the five years period of the offer the numbers would correspondingly multiply by up to five times.

Whenever I discussed the donation with officials from the countries concerned, many would register surprise. In fact, the matter was self-explanatory; many AIDS devastated countries were desperate for any help they could get and the promised 166,365 doses of Nevirapine were a life-line. If any of the forty-four nominated beneficiary countries cared to check with BI about the weight and bulk of the cargo they were to expect, in order to prepare the warehouses to store the big consignment of donated drugs, they would be surprised. The issue of storage space was not among the meticulous conditions that were set, for the simple reason that it was not necessary. Here was one instance where the notorious "infrastructure" deficiency in Africa was not an insurmountable problem. Was it somehow forgotten or was it not important? No huge cargo spaces on any ships or plane had been booked either, because each of the forty-four countries could literally have carried their share of the donated tablets as hand luggage!

The then recommended dose of Nevirapine for prevention (or more correctly reduction) of HIV virus being passed on from an infected mother to her baby was just one tablet, while her newborn child needed about half a teaspoon of the syrup of the same drug. Therefore, assuming that the announced 166,365 doses were for both the mother and child, which constituted two doses, disregarding twins, then these drugs would be enough for only 83,183 mother-baby pairs in the lucky forty-four countries. This amounted to about 2000 tablets of Nevirapine per country. The two small packages that the BI representative was photographed handing over to the minister in Congo was enough to hold all the tablets if they were taken out of their bulky packaging, and still leave plenty of room to spare. Each bottle of Nevirapine syrup for babies contains 240mls, which means that the donation was only equivalent to the volume contained in about 50 Nevirapine syrup bottles per country.

It was self evident that even BI was not taking its own donation programme very seriously. The packages of both tablets and syrup were the same commercial ones specially designed for long-term AIDS treatment in combination with other drugs. It is incredible for a company that had announced such a large donation to omit making any arrangement to offer appropriate packaging for their drugs tailored to the programme needs. For instance, for a new-born baby who needed only about 2.5 to 5 mls of the syrup, a bottle with 240mls had to be opened to get the tiny amounts out. The donation did not even include drug-dispensing kits to try and measure the tiny doses from the oversized containers. That was about the total sum of the celebrated donation.

Despite all that, the donation did not materialise everywhere it was promised, and where it did, it was not always in a timely manner. The blame for this was as usual put squarely on the shoulders of the poor countries for not having prepared the infrastructure to implement the programme. However, in this case, talk about infrastructure was just pitiful. What infrastructure was necessary for an HIV infected mother to swallow just one tablet as soon as she goes into labour, and put a few drops of syrup in her baby's mouth within seventy-two hours after birth in order to save her own baby from AIDS?

If instead of this donation, BI had just given a "no objection" to generic pharmaceutical companies to manufacture Nevirapine, cost of the entire BI donation would have at most amounted to a mere $2500 per country. Even an offer of this magnitude was not to be fully honoured.

BI set some conditions for women to qualify for access to their drugs donation. The women had to have a documented HIV positive test, attend antenatal clinics and deliver in an accredited healthcare facility under qualified medical supervision, to ensure "safe and effective use" of their drug. In most poor countries women just cannot fulfil all these conditions. One has to ask: were these very detailed measures out of concern for the safety of the women in order to protect them from the toxic effect of just one pill? Yes, just one pill. That's all each woman had to take to reduce the chance of her baby being born with the killer AIDS. This was one of the simplest treatment regimens known to modern medicine. The net effects of these measures were to ensure that only a small number of those in need would qualify.

If BI had considered the constraints serious enough to negatively impact on their own donor project then they ought to have incorporated robust components to help poor women qualify. On the contrary, no help was offered for the very basic Voluntary Testing and Counselling (VCT) of poor pregnant women. Yet it was a condition that they had to have an HIV test before they could access the drugs. Needless to say, there was no preventive programme support, no support for drugs logistics or improvement of infrastructure, which had also been identified as a major constraint. There was no effort to ease restrictions to allow the licensing or parallel importation of Nevirapine, which was already being manufactured at a much cheaper price by a number of generic manufacturers to quickly reach many more people in need. Quite the reverse, the promise of free drugs would slow down the growing market share of the more affordable generic Nevirapine, yet it was also on demand as one of the constituents of combination antiretroviral therapy. Therefore the indirect aim of the donation was to delay access to the more affordable drugs by the larger number of AIDS patients who needed Nevirapine for treatment.

In response to the announcement by Boehringer Ingelheim on July 8, 2003, activist groups immediately scoffed at BI's statement, and decried the failure to address such issues as VCT and breast-feeding as grossly unethical. They criticised the donation because it provided no structure or timetable for implementation and no details of government involvement. They predicted that this would ultimately offer very little medication for a very few people and this is precisely what happened. The activists complained that BI did not even contact other pharmaceutical companies for unified action, which would make an impact. Here, of course, the activists were totally mistaken. In terms of amount and cost, the BI donation had no major impact on the general ARV drugs cost. Therefore there was no breaking of ranks to threaten other pharmaceutical companies. The solidarity of pharmaceutical companies was holding as strong as ever, and care was taken by BI to make it abundantly clear that Nevirapine for combination ART where it was used in big amounts would continue to be sold at the usual price. This is all the rest of the big Pharma needed to know. In addition, this donation had the overarching benefit of projecting all the pharmaceutical companies in a good light. There was therefore absolutely no cause for alarm.

This donation created a big media hype, which somehow slowed down the activist pressure and competition from generic drugs without a genuine increase in access to antiretroviral therapy. In addition, it also served as an indirect demonstration that the so-called infrastructure constraints really existed in Africa. Africa's bluff was called. "Look. It is not the cost of the drugs, stupid. They can't even use the free ones."

The whole saga underscores the urgent need for Africa to look to her interests, and scrutinise every new donation. Africa must work harder towards self-sustainability starting with doing all the things they can do by and for themselves. Not all donations should be accepted all the time, because some of them end up as aid to the donor. However, to make this offer, BI was aware of the desperation of AIDS in battered Sub-Saharan Africa that was faced with the mounting deaths of her children. Indeed the gesture was in the right direction. However, if African leaders had taken time to seriously evaluate this offer they would have found that there was no single country on the continent that could not afford to buy enough Nevirapine tablets for prevention of mother to child transmission of HIV. Instead Africa should have insisted on a better donor package that also included at least treatment support for the mothers and cases of children where their own donated treatment for prevention failed. If this was not acceptable, then BI would have been asked to just allow generic copies of their patented drug which would have saved many more lives. That is if saving as many lives as possible was BI's purpose for making the donation in the first place. Many of the mothers who were offered one pill to protect their babies were themselves in advanced stages of AIDS, and desperately needed Nevirapine as part of combination therapy to save their own lives as to go on to look after their babies. Offering just one tablet to such mothers whose own lives were in mortal danger, and who would succumb to AIDS as soon as they had given birth, was morally questionable. Other than the Red Cross and Red Crescent in war situations, there are no internationally agreed ethical guidelines or standards for humanitarian interventions in disasters like AIDS. These may need to be established and monitored under international accord to cover all disasters anywhere in the world.

Despite its flaws, there is no doubt that BI was responding to a desperate humanitarian need in Africa. BI realised that their patented product Nevirapine had the power to alleviate the situation of the babies who were dying a preventable death. However, it is difficult to understand why it was not imperative for them to consider addressing important humanitarian issues like offering treatment to mothers whose children's lives they purported to save. It was obvious that the mothers who needed antiretroviral treatment for their own lives would suffer and die because they had no alternative source of life-saving therapy. It was also clear that the "rescued" babies would become orphans as a result. It was also apparent that some of the babies initially protected from HIV by Nevirapine risked acquiring the disease from their infected mothers' breast milk since they had no other source of safe food. For such affected babies, the favour that Nevirapine would do for them was simply a short stay of execution. I do not take this as a specific criticism of BI's donation but rather as a lesson for the future as conditions remain ripe for the same kind of situation to happen again.

On the other hand, while these events unfolded one would be forgiven for thinking that the drug in the centre of it all - Nevirapine - was an otherwise trouble-free medicine. On the contrary, it triggered a greater controversy than any AIDS drug to date. It also highlighted yet another kind of dilemma faced by poor patients and scientists working in resource-constrained countries trying to find remedies for disastrous diseases, especially when the West funds the involved research. As detailed below, it often entails being caught between a rock and a hard place.

The Nevirapine Crisis

Although highly effective therapy for prevention of mother to child HIV transmission was well known and had by mid 1990s been established as a standard of care in the West, it remained inaccessible in Sub-Saharan Africa because it was unaffordable. This left poor pregnant HIV infected African women without any treatment to save their babies - even by as late as the year 2000. These wretched women were left with no alternative but to choose between the horrible and the terrible. Either they had to undergo a risky back street abortion (since abortion is illegal in almost all African countries), or, resign themselves to the nightmare of giving birth to a baby with strong likelihood of being HIV infected, and the dire consequences that go with it.

Throughout the 1990s, a huge number of African HIV-infected children died as we, the healthcare providers, watched without any therapy to offer. Relentlessly, the death of little babies due to AIDS mounted year after year with no end in sight. Needless to say, even the small numbers of HIV infected babies that somehow survived early death were still doomed to die later, and no less excruciatingly as they too had no access to antiretroviral therapy. Meanwhile the magnitude of the crisis was underscored by the tragic fact that an estimated one million children were being infected with perinatal HIV every year in poor countries.

The most painful aspect of childhood AIDS was the torture due to horrific infections, which the little ones had to endure before their inevitable demise. Any healthcare provider unfortunate enough to have witnessed this (and this was virtually everyone working in Uganda and most of Sub-Saharan Africa) never forgot it. As there was no foreseeable prospect of the cost of drugs coming down, Africa just

braced for more agony. In such dire circumstances, the critical need
for any intervention, which could alleviate the situation in some way,
was imperative. Africa just needed something done urgently to avert
further genocide. Meanwhile, no action was forthcoming from the rich
world that could have put a stop to the misery.

In the midst of this gloom some light of hope was lit. Some Ugandan
and American scientists, including Francis Mmiro, Brooks Jackson
and Laura Guay from Johns Hopkins University in USA, tried to find
a practical solution to alleviate this tragic situation. Jackson and Guay
were eyewitnesses to the catastrophe of AIDS during their many
years of working with us in Uganda. The drug chosen for study was
Nevirapine because some background knowledge about it suggested
that it had a good chance of reducing the transmission of HIV from
an infected pregnant woman passing to her baby. A single dose of
Nevirapine was already known to stay effective against HIV in the body
for over 48 hours, and to be safe for both the mother and baby. Therefore
they set out to determine whether Nevirapine could be used to save at
least some of the doomed babies. If this treatment, which involved just
one pill for the mother and one small teaspoonful of the same medicine
in syrup form for the baby, was found to be efficacious, it would be a
breakthrough for any resource-constrained country like Uganda. The
alternative treatment used in rich countries was unaffordable because
it involved an expensive combination of antiretroviral drugs which
needed to be used daily for a long period. In addition, the women on
treatment were monitored with expensive laboratory tests to ensure
safety.

The novel research was designed to find an affordable alternative
tailored to poor conditions. Naturally, the besieged Ugandan
healthcare providers readily supported the research proposal because
it promised to find a way out of their daily anguish. All Ugandan
research regulatory bodies also unanimously endorsed it after very
careful review. The United States National Institute of Health (NIH)
was approached to provide funding for the study. The proposal had to
undergo tough ethical and scientific review before NIH could decide
whether to provide the funds or not. Once again, the clear scientific

merit of the proposed study, and especially the potential to save many Ugandan lives, carried the day.

The study finally got under way in 1997, and involved 645 mother-infant pairs. It proceeded very well and was completed according to schedule. The earnestly awaited results were published in September 1999 and the findings caused excitement in Uganda, and indeed in most resource constrained countries. The findings promised the very first affordable and easily applicable life-saving ART for poor countries. Basically, the results clearly demonstrated that just a single dose of Nevirapine given to the mother and a single dose to the infant significantly reduced HIV transmission from an infected mother to her child. Furthermore, it had the added advantage that it could still work even when the mother had little or no antenatal care. Many mothers in many poor countries often turned up for the very first time at healthcare facilities while in labour. Even if such women were not HIV tested but were merely diagnosed on the basis of a suggestive history or clinical signs of HIV, the treatment would still be effective. The therapy also had a good safety profile. In case it was mistakenly given to a non-infected mother, the tiny dose would do no harm. Clearly, this discovery was an important breakthrough for Prevention of Mother to Child Transmission (PMTCT) of HIV in poor countries. For the very first time Africa had a treatment option that could be used to lessen the carnage of AIDS. It was this landmark research that provided the scientific basis for the controversial Boehringer Ingelheim Nevirapine donation.

Just as the poor countries scrambled to prepare their antenatal clinics in order to expand the use of Nevirapine for PMTCT programmes, and to meet BI's conditions, which included setting up makeshift facilities, ready to take advantage of the donation, things fell apart. It looked like Africa just could not win! The flashpoint of the controversy was across the oceans in the United States following the publication of the study results. There, the use of the Nevirapine model for prevention of mother to child transmission of HIV came under severe criticism. Though it had all started rather insidiously, by March 2002, new concerns were raised with regard to the conduct of the study and NIH, the study sponsor, was forced to hold special sessions to investigate the matter.

Unremittingly, the Nevirapine saga had by the following year exploded into an international media storm.

The highly publicised controversy could be traced back to NIH. It seems to have had its origin in a dispute between Dr Jonathan M. Fishbein, the former director of the Office of Policy in Research Operations at the U.S. National Institute of Allergy and Infectious Diseases (NIAID), in the National Institutes of Health (NIH) of United States, and his supervisors. Dr. Fishbein was reportedly hired by NIH in July 2003, and was informed just over six months later that he would be dismissed. The doctor allegedly responded in fighting mood. He sought whistleblower protection and made allegations against his employer, NIAID, which he accused of gross "scientific and professional misconduct." Later in a detailed forty-three page document, Dr. Fishbein admonished the conduct and results of the study. Among the deficiencies he cited were insufficient staff, poor organisation of critical source documents and insufficient standard operating procedures (SOPs), which he alleged had compromised patient safety. In a presentation to the National Academy of Sciences, he accused NIH of "failure to comply with mandatory health and safety requirements in AIDS-research programmes."

On our side, in the midst of AIDS devastation, this astounding controversy was clearly a double-edged sword. The most important issue in 1999 was not that Nevirapine was the best option for PMTCT, but rather that it was the only practicable choice available to the poor. Nevirapine, its shortcomings not withstanding, had the potential to save up to half of the babies who would otherwise have got infected with AIDS and died. However, some people argued relentlessly that the study did not meet US standards. This may be true as far as the strict details of the scientific protocol were concerned, and as far as it applied to US conditions. However, as far as we were concerned, in the midst of a tragic emergency in Africa, this point of view appeared to be either myopic or callous. It brought into focus some very important issues that have dogged research funding from the rich countries in favour of the poor ones. What standards of research should be adopted, and whose regulations should be followed? The rich countries are endowed with state-of-the-art facilities, and have all the manpower and advanced technology to meet the highest standards possible. If research requirements insisted on such standards and facilities, it would straight away deny research opportunities to the poor, and with it the ability to prioritise their own agenda aimed at addressing their own issues. Therefore, the pertinent question was whether the current US Good Clinical Practice standards are always appropriate or applicable for research in developing countries, for which they were not designed. The main criticism of the Nevirapine study was that the US guidelines were not always followed in detail in the trial. "Thousands" of times screamed Dr. Fishbein's damning report.

The vital question here was: could the same research objectives and patient protection be achieved in a variety of settings and using different approaches without compromising the critical standards necessary to make the study scientifically valid? If the answer is not "Yes" then there is a very serious problem. In this case, the study was harshly judged by US criteria which did not always apply to Uganda. One particular area that came in for sharp criticism by Dr. Fishbein was the reporting of adverse events, especially serious ones. The NIAID research definitions of serious adverse events covered events beyond those considered serious or relevant by the Ugandan researchers. Furthermore, he took exception to the fact that the Americans did not formally authorise some modifications that were necessitated by this situation. These were some of the issues that he considered vitally important to bring up. A counter argument by John S. James in his article about the same subject published in *AIDS Treatment News*, December 2004, throws more light on this issue:

> A strong case could be made that imposing the same research requirements regardless of infrastructure and environment can result in second-class standards for developing countries ... Instead of fighting over how strictly to enforce rules that are sometimes unworkable, why not design rules that will better protect people and data, while helping staff get their work done correctly?

It is amazing that the issue of US standards arose with regard to this vital study for Africa. In such circumstances, it would be justified to ask whether the rich countries would be magnanimous enough to undertake all the research for all diseases that affect the poor even if their own people were not affected? In this case the USA just did not have this devastating catastrophe running riot in their midst. If they had such an emergency, you can be sure that the reaction would have been vigorous. The reality was that mother-to-child transmission of HIV had almost been wiped out in the USA. This followed the discovery and widespread use of a more robust ART regimen, which, unlike poor countries like Uganda, they could comfortably afford. Yet it was Africa that was now bleeding and in urgent need of an affordable life-saving alternative. Devastated Sub-Saharan Africa could not afford the American standard of care for its poor patients. Virtually all donors had not responded to the plight of millions of poor HIV infected pregnant mothers in desperate need of emergency help. Obviously, the contentious Nevirapine study in Uganda was not in any way aiming to produce a medication that could ever be considered for use in USA for the simple reason that USA already had a much superior alternative. Why was it then critically necessary to insist on application of strict American standards in order to produce a drug that could not possibly meet the US standards nor be acceptable for use in the USA? Why? Even if the USA, in a sudden rush of overwhelming charity, decided to put its own citizens on the line to carry out a state-of-the-art study on behalf of poor African HIV infected women, it would have met with formidable ethical barriers. Questions would immediately arise whether it is acceptable for the US to carry out a study to determine an inferior outcome for the poor countries. Even if these obstacles were somehow overcome, the USA would still not have come under great pressure to prioritise the study or to act with the uttermost urgency that the situation demanded. During my long practice as a researcher and AIDS physician, this unfair state of affairs has saddened me often. This is the same kind of weird reasoning that has so often been used to deny our people care and life-saving interventions. Millions in Africa have been left to die as a result. Excuses have been given, interspersed with belated apologies, when all that was required was sensible humanitarian action. When Africa took the initiative (in partnership with experts from the developed countries) in the most appropriate way possible, trying to find a solution to this devastating carnage which the world had ignored – see what happened.

Even the hardened critics of the study conceded that the slight differences in research methodology did not change the validity of the findings and the scientific conclusions. When all misplaced entries and the few missing data in some case notes were taken into account, still the study outcome remained unaffected. Considering its importance, the study should have been highly commended for the milestone discovery of an intervention that had the potential to save hundreds of thousands of lives at the time when the poor had no alternative.

The controversy notwithstanding, the Nevirapine study demonstrated innovative research that addressed a critical public issue, and ensured a very low drop-out and excellent follow-up. Overall, the mother and infant pair follow-up for the first six weeks was an impressive 97.4 %. Yet the negative publicity so scared would-be users of this good treatment, and, almost certainly, some babies who could have been saved died as this misguided debate raged. For instance, in a press release on July 28, 2003, the South African Medicines Control Council announced that Nevirapine would be rejected as a single agent in reducing the transmission of HIV from mother to child in their country, citing the controversy as the reason. Yet they did not immediately implement a superior substitute. I gathered later that even the whistleblower who raised the alarm also acknowledge that the results of the study were important. However, I did not hear any expression of disquiet for the dying babies, especially those who may have died because of concerns about the drug that the controversy raised. I did not hear of any suggestions for an alternative, or any appeal for affordable life saving drugs like those in use in USA.

I found it perplexing that anyone would disagree with the scientists and funding agencies who responded to a truly humanitarian crisis in an effort to find a relief. This is not to say that relief projects or studies could not be criticised. Constructive criticism is good for any study and is always welcome. Although the safety of participants is paramount in any ethical study, it does not mean that it must be ensured unvaryingly always in all situations. For instance, hospitalisation of a research subject for any cause is taken as a serious event in research in the USA. However, criteria for hospitalisation in the USA vary from that of Uganda. For instance, in Uganda patients suffering from some endemic diseases are usually treated as outpatients, and chronic lack of hospital beds determines the level of seriousness of the illness as a criterion for admission. In research, the objective and expected outcomes may be different in different situations. Nevirapine, though inferior to the American standard, was preferable to nothing since it could save many of the babies that would otherwise have been infected and died. It was especially valid in Uganda because it was tailored to the Ugandan situation. The variations to the US approach were not relevant as long as the science was right and the participants lives were not put at any risk.

However, this does not mean that the poor are in any way happy with the second best in healthcare. It is only poverty that has boxed them in. This inequitable state of affairs will remain a gross embarrassment to the world. Clearly, the ultimate goal should be the best standard of healthcare for everybody. Unfortunately, the reality is that this criterion is a long way from being attained. It has not even been given the kind of priority consideration that it deserves as a crucial world equity issue.

5

Gunning for a Solution

Taking the Bull by the Horns

Towards the end of the 1990s, the deaths continued to mount in Uganda and the whole of Sub-Saharan Africa. Yet some people thought that the worst that could happen had already come to pass and therefore there was just no more room for the situation to deteriorate further. They were grossly mistaken. While it was true that the numbers of new infections had sharply declined in Uganda, the huge numbers already infected and those coming down with full blown AIDS were on a sharp rise. This rise and the mounting deaths corresponded proportionally with the numbers in desperate need of antiretroviral therapy. Yet most patients were too poor to afford the life-saving drugs. Each day in my clinic seemed to be worse than the previous one. New and old cases endlessly turned up, each one hoping against hope that somehow I could invoke some magic to whisk them out of their terrifying situation.

My long experience working among AIDS patients had taught me to spot diagnose at a glance many of the common opportunistic infections which AIDS patients commonly presented. As I strolled through the waiting room full of patients I could immediately spot that the one covering her head had been hit by an attack of shingles on her face. The other one breathing fast as if there was no oxygen in the room had Pneumocystis Pneumonia (PCP). I could see that the man with his hands wrapped around his head, as if it was a heavy delicate glass that had to be protected from accidental fall, had Cryptococcus Meningitis; while the sick-looking but incongruously happy, talkative man had HIV psychosis. I could see many others whose secondary diagnoses were quite obvious to me as evidenced by such signs as eczematous skin eruptions, inflamed lips with white-coated inner edges, and shrivelled bodies. Some others presented other more easily recognisable AIDS associated signs that were known by virtually everyone else in the community. However, for the majority of my patients their most serious tormentor was not the external manifestations of AIDS or the physical pain that they so obviously endured. It was psychological agony.

The new patients were usually in the most urgent need of psychological support because they were the most distraught. Their problems were more varied than the old cases. Very few diseases manifest as many varied physical and psychosomatic problems as does AIDS. The main reason why the old cases were calmer was because they would have been through the "AIDS cycle" of events that started on the very first day when the grim diagnosis was made. At the beginning they would have suffered the shock of discovering that they were infected with HIV. This would be followed by blame in a futile attempt to put the cause of their insufferable problem on the shoulders of someone else. Next, they would lapse into a state of denial - deluding themselves that somehow the whole thing was just a bad dream. Thus, some patients would attribute their plight to witchcraft, while others would think that they suffered from other less frightening diseases. Others would believe that they were merely victims of laboratory errors. For a while many would try to distance themselves from reality, by deceiving themselves that they were not really infected. But the unforgiving virus would wear them down regardless, because it would keep on multiplying fast - billions of times every day while destroying billions of cells in the process as the victim weakened, inevitably forcing the sufferer to eventually come face to face with the monster. The relatives of those blinded by stigma or denial would worry on their behalf. Then, frantically, the sufferers would finally seek to escape, but, realising that there was just no way out, they would just sit and wait for death. Often they did not have to wait long.

Some relatives accompanying patients to my clinic often requested to have a private word with me before the patient was brought in. "Doctor, we have been through hell to get him here," was a common whisper from many fearful relatives. "We think he has AIDS, because he lost his wife a year ago. Please help us to get him to accept his condition and save his life." There was hardly any need to mention the cause of death. It was only if one died of some other cause that it was usually mentioned, often not for the purpose of setting the record straight but rather for denying that it was AIDS. Many patients already suspected or knew that they had AIDS, but chose to keep it a tightly guarded secret because of the stigma, or because they just wanted to spare their relatives the pain or hide the "shame" of it all. Many were not as scared of death as they were of the pain and disfigurement the disease would cause them before the inevitable happened.

Suffering and deaths increased all the time throughout the 1990s. It was a nightmare experience for all HIV/AIDS care providers in Sub-Saharan Africa and much more so for the families of the victims. Meanwhile, people talked incessantly about the new anti-AIDS drugs, which were saving the lives of American and European AIDS patients. In Uganda virtually everyone knew about the work of the Joint Clinical Research Centre in increasing access to the newly-discovered AIDS drugs. By the end of 1997 it was already common knowledge that the JCRC was successfully treating a large number of patients with Highly Active Antiretroviral Therapy (HAART). HAART, also known as ART, was whispered to be a "miraculous cure." At the time, the JCRC was one of the biggest providers of ART in Africa, if not the biggest. Thousands of desperate patients flocked to the centre including a sizeable number from all neighbouring countries. There were even a few that came in from as far away as the Democratic Republic of Congo, Malawi, Ethiopia, and even war-torn Liberia. But all these patients were either very rich or had benefactors to pay the exorbitant price of their AIDS drugs. Sadly, most of those who rushed to the JCRC for the magical pills met only with disappointment. They found the price above their means. Instead, many had to settle for the highly hyped up poor man's AIDS drug, the cheap Cotrimoxazole (Septrin/Bactrim) prophylaxis as they braced for more suffering. Many had nothing else to do but try out numerous herbal and Western drug concoctions - which were uniformly useless - as they awaited the inevitable. Many patients told me that the most heart-wrenching agony they suffered was partly to do with being aware that life-saving therapy did indeed exist but was not available to them, only because they were poor. To them, the actual cause of their looming death was no longer the dreadful AIDS but poverty and denial. Meanwhile, we the care providers on the frontline had nothing to offer except our shoulders for the poor patients to cry on. We were the big Pharma's involuntary proxy "fall guys" who apologised to the patients and bore their wrath and frustration on their behalf. Meanwhile, the pharmaceutical companies were laughing all the way to the top of the stock exchange market.

Meanwhile in the southernmost part of the African continent events were unfolding that would bring people out onto the streets in worldwide protests. Despite being in a state of denial at the time, the government of AIDS-ridden South Africa, which had most of the world's AIDS sufferers (then estimated at over 4.5 million), was facing pressure to immediately start providing lifesaving therapy to their suffering citizens. Over 400,000 were estimated to have already died, and without therapy at least a fifth of all AIDS sufferers would die within a decade. Although South Africa is the richest country on the continent, she still found the cost of drugs too exorbitant. One year's therapy was then priced in excess of $6,000, but with generic versions the cost could be dramatically reduced to less than a tenth of that. Use of generic antiretroviral drugs was highly successful in increasing accessibility to ARVs, and therefore made nationwide AIDS treatment programmes possible. For instance, and most impressively too, when the Brazilian government, which was at about the same economic level as South Africa, began to manufacture generic copies of AIDS drugs in 1998, the cost fell by an average of 79 %, thus making it possible to provide her citizens with universal free treatment. This was soon followed by further good news for Brazilians. There was a resultant drastic fall of over 50 % in the death rate due to AIDS.

When South Africa, with a more serious problem than Brazil, belatedly and reluctantly started considering the use of lower cost generic copies, by invoking a 1997 law that allowed their importation and use, all hell broke loose. On March 5, 2001, the local Pharmaceutical Manufacturers' Association and thirty-nine rapacious pharmaceutical companies dragged the South African government to the courts of law in Pretoria for patents infringement. All pharmaceutical companies were mobilised to demonstrate solidarity and speak with one loud voice so that their resolve could not be doubted. As a unitary group they were in a better position to fight off the inevitable condemnation of this cold-hearted action which ignored the plight of poor South Africans in the face of this undeniable human tragedy.

The big Pharma cannot have expected the South African government to put up a spirited fight in court. At the time, the government was not even officially convinced that AIDS was actually caused by HIV! A highly controversial debate was raging in the country about the efficacy of antiretroviral drugs. Therefore, the Pharmaceutical companies cannot have expected that this government which was in denial would suddenly turn round and challenge them in courts of law seeking to make these same drugs accessible. However, by allowing the situation to get to this level of brinkmanship, both the South African government and the Big Pharma had walked themselves into a sticky situation, from which they could not easily extricate themselves. Before either side blinked, the show was snatched out of their hands by the human rights organisations and activists. Then the whole affair unfolded into a major international news story that exposed what was described as the greed of the big Pharma and the ineptness of the South African government in the face of the AIDS catastrophe, causing both of them great embarrassment. The commercial stakes were higher on the big Pharma's side and they could not allow South Africa to get away Scot-free because this would set a precedent, and become an ominous threat to their monopoly and profits.

While South Africa was busy fighting it out with the pharmaceutical companies in the law courts in Pretoria, amid unprecedented protests and demonstrations, almost two thousand kilometres north in Uganda, and more specifically at the JCRC, I was also involved in a quiet but no less serious battle with both the pharmaceutical companies and our own National Drugs Authority (NDA). My struggle, however, did not make it to the headlines and this was just as well. What triggered the radical measures that I took was the need to find a way to alleviate the disturbing daily carnage caused by AIDS, and to answer desperate appeals by our patients' demands for life-saving AIDS drugs. I was even beginning to be scared of answering my own telephone, as incessant AIDS patients in search of treatment never gave me any reprieve. I was tired of making endless apologies to dying patients when I knew very well that generic manufacturers in Brazil, India, and an increasing number of other countries were manufacturing the antiretroviral drugs cheaply. However, the Trade Related Aspects of Intellectual Property Rights (TRIPS) and patents laws, policed by the World Trade Organisation (WTO), restricted access to them.

Despite the highly charged atmosphere and the seemingly insurmountable problems, I felt that I had no alternative but to try and bring in the more affordable generic AIDS drugs for my desperate patients. I recall asking myself how many deaths it was going to take for the world to appreciate that too many people had died. I could see no help on the way. I decided not to involve anyone else, as the move I was about to take was not without risk. Without breathing a word to the awesome Uganda National Drugs Authority, I just placed an order for the generic AIDS drugs from the Cipla pharmaceutical company of India. In so doing I was under no illusion that I could just get away with it. I was, however, prepared for the worst. But I felt that I had to respond to the outcry of the numerous desperate patients who flocked to me daily. This was a moral dilemma. I could no longer bear the sight of so many people continuing to die a preventable death while I stood by. I felt strongly that if I failed to act on behalf of my patients then I would be in breach of my professional commitment to save lives. It was not that I was not afraid of the consequences of my action, including imprisonment, but rather I was more horrified by the suffering of my patients. This went against my otherwise peaceful and non-confrontational inclination, not to mention my detestation of acting contrary to the law. However, as many who know me well can testify, if there is a justifiable humanitarian cause consistent with my professional calling to save lives, I am never to be found wanting.

Many have asked me why I did not patiently wait and follow the correct channels. Obviously this would have been most unwise considering the prevailing adverse circumstances. Mere bureaucratic procedures would have condemned the initiative as a non-starter. The

NDA would have read me clauses from their small book pointing out that importation of new drugs required long, exhaustive procedures, including testing for purity and efficacy prior to their registration, and this could take years. The Ugandan government would have been unwise to authorise the importation of the same kind of drugs that had landed the more powerful South African government in the dock. I think, at the very best, the most sympathetic response I could have expected from our government would have been a recommendation that I await the resolution of the South African case first.

As the head of the biggest AIDS research and treatment centre in Africa, not many other people were under as much pressure from desperate patients as I was. On an almost daily basis, I came face-to-face with the unbearable pain of AIDS-infected orphans and vulnerable children to whom I had nothing to offer. I witnessed the anguish of their caretakers and parents, as their beloved children succumbed to the Grim Reaper. I took deep breaths just to keep calm as I saw the desperation of wailing and tearful children watching as their parents died. I was the one who heard the confessions of desperate AIDS victims who considered murdering their loved ones instead of leaving them to suffer the torture of AIDS. I witnessed with shock the suicides of those who could not take it anymore, and the endless torture and deaths of the different but invariably painful end that befell the youths in our society as a result of AIDS. I was the one that desperate patients vented their misery, frustration and anger on. It was I that desperate relatives called to the deathbeds of their loved ones. I could do nothing to stop more and more patients who kept coming. If I tried to rest my mind a little, then the likes of Paulo would rudely remind me. There was no escape. The problem had either to be endured or addressed. If this was not justification enough to take the bull by the horns then I do not know a better one. Obviously, if the Government, and more specifically the NDA, had suspected my intention to import generic antiretroviral drugs, they would have taken prompt action.

When Cipla received my order in their offices in Mumbai, it was not with as much enthusiasm as would have been expected of a company about to make their first major lucrative business deal. The killjoy was the international patents law and TRIPS agreement. Cipla insisted on guarantees that I would take full responsibility and shoulder any repercussions and lawsuits that might follow. I immediately wrote back assuring them that I would take the responsibility. In reality, however, this was just hot air. How could I have been expected to give such guarantees? I was just a simple doctor, and not even a significant government official. All that I had to give as a guarantee was perhaps my neck. It's all I had. Therefore my assurances were not worth the electronic micro byte it was conveyed on. Incredibly Cipla was reassured enough to process the order. The consignment of drugs was airlifted to Entebbe airport to be immediately impounded on arrival by both Customs and the stunned NDA officials, just as I expected. Then the crisis began as I braced for the worst.

Predictably the immediate reaction of NDA was to have me arrested and prosecuted for importation of unauthorised drugs in direct contravention of established regulations, and secondly to send back the drugs at my expense. A quick check revealed that I had neither used government nor donor money for the purchase of the drugs. All the funds had been raised by an innovative savings scheme that I had set up at the JCRC to raise funds from service charges paid by private clients of the centre. Absence of a third party involvement made it easier for the NDA to take castigatory action and they made it clear that they intended to let loose the full force of the law against me. I explained that I had an obligation to the thousands of patients who besieged me in a desperate bid to save their lives. This was the primary reason that I was employed by the JCRC: This cut no ice with them. However, on my side, I was in no doubt that in the dire circumstances, I had done the best that I possibly could to try and save lives of at least some Ugandans. The ball was now in the NDA's court, and it was up to them to do their job by finding ways and means to allow the drugs into the country even if it included locking me up as a scapegoat.

Meanwhile, a few local journalists and some patients got wind of an interesting story involving the barring of life-saving drugs by the NDA at the airport, and started asking questions. The drugs had truly brought things to a head as I had hoped and prayed. Word reached the corridors of power and a crisis meeting was called in the President's office involving cabinet ministers, the NDA, Ministry of Health officials and some legal experts. The NDA put up a spirited case against me informing the meeting that my action was a blatant breach of the law, which needed an appropriate punitive action. I did not try to deny the charges because the NDA representative who led the "prosecution" was not doing it out of malice. He was merely a typical robotic civil service technocrat, just doing his job. I simply explained that all the people attending the meeting including myself had relatives with AIDS who were tormenting me with their frantic requests for the life-saving therapy. I explained that the available drugs were too expensive, and as a result people were dying a preventable death. I had therefore taken action, to save lives, as any other responsible doctor would have done. "I did not try to smuggle the drugs in but presented them to legal official channels for clearance," I pleaded. "What remains is for you to take a decision whether to allow them in or not." I concluded.

The genial chairman, Dr Ruhakana Rugunda, the Minister for the Presidency, and the others present were not too difficult to convince as the scourge of AIDS had bitten hard on all Ugandans. Also, the government and especially the President were very much in support of AIDS alleviation measures, and therefore it was politically correct for politicians to be seen to toe this line. For that reason the mood of the meeting was quickly shifting from throwing me into jail to finding a way to clear the drugs. The NDA chairman and lawyers at the meeting were requested to take a good look at the regulations and see if there was a loop hole or any clause under which the drugs could possibly be allowed into the country legally. "Yes, indeed there is," the legal officer said after a quick scan of the statute. "The emergency clause covers this," he added. This to me sounded like music!

"There is your reprieve, Mugyenyi. You may clear your drugs out of the airport but in future make absolutely sure that you follow the NDA regulations." I was warned. However, I could see that many were delighted and relieved that the drugs had been cleared. The most notable exception was me! "Sir, I would like to first of all apologise for not following the set procedure, but I am sorry I cannot accept your offer to let the drugs in," I said to the stunned meeting.

"Now what is the problem, my brother Peter?" asked the amazed chairman.

"Sir, AIDS treatment is for life! If you only allow this consignment in you will be postponing the patients' deaths for only a little while. I would like reassurances that all subsequent consignments will not be barred," I replied.

"Dr Mugyenyi. You are a trickster, aren't you?" one NDA officer close to me retorted.

"No, it makes perfect sense," a member on the other side came to my defence. "And the same clause can always apply with follow-up shipments."

"Thatta boy!" I remarked.

Members did not realise at the time that they had just made a historic decision which, besides saving thousands of Ugandan lives, would also have repercussions the world over. Two important events in quick succession followed the release of the drugs from the airport. The most important result was that the numbers of patients who for the first time could afford the ARVs increased so much so that I made the second order for a much bigger consignment almost immediately. Secondly, a week or so later, I got two unexpected visitors. They introduced themselves as "somehow connected with the pharmaceutical industry that had taken the South African government to court." They said that they were just in the neighbourhood, and had dropped in for a brief chat, without being more specific. For the first time I met people connected with pharmaceutical companies who did not flash out glossy visiting cards and brochures, or make out embellished pleasantries legendary of drugs salesmen. They came straight to the point. "We understand that you started importing generic ARV drugs." I answered in the affirmative. "Are you aware that there is a court case going on in South Africa for infringement of the international patents' law with regard to the use of the same drugs?"

"Yes, I am very much aware and I follow the progress of the case regularly" I replied as coolly as possible, but not without a little anxiety.

"We are not here to make any kind of unpleasant threats, but this does not look like a wise move at this crucial time. Why did you do it?"

The part about not making threats was certainly welcome. I had feared that things could get nasty. It was quite clear from their unsmiling faces that they had not come to humour me.

"Sorry, I did not set out to break any rules but I face dying patients on a daily basis. I thought I could make a difference by bringing in drugs that at least some of our people could afford - I mean drugs that could save their lives and alleviate their agony," I answered truthfully.

"Cost is your problem?"

"It is the main constraint."

"Well, we fully appreciate your position and would like to help," one of them said.

"Thank you," I said hardly disguising my surprise that these men would be so understanding! However, considering that they had been hesitant to declare their affiliations, I kept up my guard.

"Tell us how much you paid for the drugs and, for you only, we shall match it."

I showed them the invoices and they confirmed that they would indeed offer me the same cost.

"Now you have no reason to import the copies anymore, do you?"

"Absolutely not, as long as the price is either the same or lower," I replied enthusiastically, but not immediately grasping the full implication of their offer. But momentarily, I saw this offer was different, and not the usual "circus" as I felt a surge of excitement. This was a historic moment. For the first time in my long struggle to find AIDS drugs for our people, I could see a glimmer of hope for our long-suffering patients. I began to visualise a breakthrough. With immediate effect, our middle-income group would no longer die needlessly! My mind even started drifting towards universal access to ART, which only a week earlier had been just inconceivable. However, I was still sober enough to realise that this was a very long way off. But, to me it was always the only target that I aimed at for our suffering people.

As soon as these bearers of the good news were out of my office, I was on the line explaining to the surprised Cipla staff in India that I would no long import drugs from them because we had been presented with a better offer from the brand manufacturers.

"We shall lower our price," was the melodious reply from Cipla.

"Now you are talking," I said to myself! This was turning out to be the best day since my AIDS career started. Though they did not know it then, a competition between the brand manufacturers and their generic counterparts had begun. The two were talking to and haggling with each other at that brief moment through me. From that day the cost of the common first line AIDS drugs was never the same, though other means of denying access by the ever-resourceful big Pharma were to emerge later.

Soon more good news followed. The pharmaceutical companies were withdrawing the court case against South Africa. That too was a great day for me, but it was followed by really disheartening news. Incredibly, the South African Government was not going to press its advantage in victory and go a step further to announce free and unhindered access to the life-saving cost effective drugs. What a difference it would have made. On the contrary, it was the denial business as usual.

I consider that people are making a mistake if they refer to either brand or generics manufacturers as being good or bad, or one better than the other. I regard both of them appropriately as "for profit" organisations whose paramount goal is to make as much money as they possibly can. They are certainly not humanitarian organisations. As one combatant big Pharma boss once put it, "We are not the Red Cross!" Both of them respond best to requests for lower prices if they are challenged by competition. I was to capitalise on this strategy many times to get further reduction and to put record numbers of patients on therapy. However, even as late as April 2005, I found that one must keep one's eyes wide open as there is always a card up their sleeve. For instance, while scrutinising the ART drugs supply bids I found that one generic manufacturer quoted a much lower price for their products to another AIDS treatment programme than that being offered to us. Asked why this was the case, the company said that the orders from our programme were for a smaller volume. Confronted with data that showed that the opposite was actually true, their answer was that they would look into it. When they finally lowered the price they increased the flight and handling charges. They only came round when I threatened to hit them where it hurts most - in their pocket - by importing drugs from other generic manufacturers.

Sadly, even with this initiative, which enabled thousands of patients to access antiretroviral therapy in Uganda, the majority of the patients still could not afford even the price of generic drugs. Therefore, the struggle was not yet won, and the challenge that still lay ahead was much more difficult than those which had been met.

Survival of the Most Competitive

A glimmer of hope that something substantial might finally be done about the AIDS scourge in poor countries originated from the G8 meeting held in Okinawa, Japan in July 2000. On their agenda for the very first time was the "urgent [though it should have read 'long denied'] need" for increased funding to poor countries to alleviate the AIDS catastrophe. This was the kind of meeting that should have taken place at least a decade earlier. The news found the people in AIDS devastated countries of Sub-Saharan Africa, engulfed in the midst of the then well established crisis, on the verge of despair thinking that the world had forsaken them. The good news lifted up the sunken spirits of both patients and care providers in the AIDS battered countries, creating cautious optimism that help would soon be on the way. All were very grateful that at least some talking was taking place even though it was very late, because it was already clear that without international intervention, the massacre would degenerate into scorched earth devastation.

During the follow-on meeting involving the African heads of states in Abuja, Nigeria, held in April 2001, attended by no less than Kofi Annan, the UN Secretary General, a call for the establishment of Global AIDS

Fund (GAF) to channel funds to fight the disease was made. This was the most exciting news to reach the terrified AIDS patients and their families since the outbreak of the epidemic, and promised to be the most serious international AIDS relief programme so far. Subsequently, a United Nations General Assembly special session on AIDS, held June 2001 ,endorsed the proposal, to be managed by an independent secretariat supported by WHO and UNAIDS. After the usual bureaucratic delay, which was so frustrating to the impatiently expectant AIDS devastated countries, the secretariat was finally established in January 2002 - almost two years after Okinawa. However, it appeared that the commitment of rich countries was to say the least half-hearted. For instance, at the initial assessment, it was conservatively estimated that to be effective the fund needed at least $7 billion immediately. However, the USA initially offered only $200 million, while France committed only $150 million. Most disappointingly, hardly any country acted with the kind of urgency that the tragic situation demanded to bring in even their meagre contributions. Sadly, but perhaps not surprisingly, the initiative that started on a high note began to falter, promising far too little for the millions who were in dire need of the life-saving drugs. It meant that too many people would still die long before the programme ever got underway because of the usual red tape. Considering the initial responses it appeared that even the programme's very best outcome would still leave many people dying because the expected funds were grossly deficient for the enormity of the crisis. However, at that time when good news for AIDS sufferers in Africa was virtually unknown, this initiative was all the hope that the patients and their families had to cling on to. As the undertaking was a worldwide effort, all nations, rich or poor, were invited to make pledges.

As the pledges trickled in, I began to evaluate the initiative in terms of lives that would be saved according to the declared pledges, but I kept coming up with very disheartening numbers. Yet many of my poor AIDS patients were bubbling with expectation that their ordeal would soon end. Many of my fellow healthcare providers thought that watching helplessly as their AIDS patients died would soon be a thing of the past. Meanwhile, the besieged UNAIDS and WHO that had shouldered much of the criticism made sure that the good news was spread quickly and widely through carefully worded press releases beamed worldwide through both print and electronic media. In Sub-Saharan Africa one could have heard sighs of relief. "At long last," so it appeared, "help was on the way."

The following year, on World AIDS Day 2003, UNAIDS and WHO announced plans to reach three million people living with AIDS in developing countries by the end of 2005, which became known as the "3 by 5 initiative." This was declared a "vital step towards the ultimate goal of providing universal access to AIDS treatment to all those who need it." The set targets, however, were absurdly low considering the much larger numbers who were left out of the equation, and in individual countries the national targets were very miserable. It was obvious that the initiative would only reach a small minority of those in need. The initiative was quiet about the fate of the majority who could not be reached and yet were equally desperate for the life-saving therapy. Notwithstanding this, the WHO bandwagon hit the road advertising the new initiative. My concern was whether the bureaucratic WHO and UNAIDS could make this an exception and deliver on their own commitment, or was this the usual media hype? On the other hand, if they failed to meet expectations, as I feared, I hoped that at least this time round we would be spared the hackneyed excuses of the so-called "constraints."

Rapidly assembled expert committees were identified and invited to Geneva to work out the details of the project, including drugs choices, treatment guidelines, and logistical requirements. Countries were facilitated to also present their own country specific recommendations and guidelines for the use of ART. Each country scrambled their own technical committees facilitated by an army of consultants who in most cases had never done this kind of work before, for the simple reason that nothing of the sort had ever happened. The WHO recommendations were good enough for any country to use, until perhaps much later when the need to fine-tune the programme would arise, if at all. The need for countries to present their own recommendations was made to look like a critical prerequisite, purportedly to promote among other things "country ownership." This was nonsense to me as it meant delaying the start of the programme, bearing in mind that it was a state of emergency.

After all, the drug choices at the time were very limited as there were only two possible choices for the first line combination drugs ready for use in poor countries. Only one was immediately accessible for wider use. In reality, therefore, there was no practical choice to make. The second option included the drug Efavirenz, then not widely available, but which was to be used in special circumstances including patients co-infected with both TB and HIV who needed therapy for both diseases at the same time. Pointlessly, the countries were kept busy chasing their own tails and, just for good measure, the exercise was further extended to include working out the second line drugs to be used if the first line drugs failed. Yet the GAF had no immediate plans or funds to buy the second line drugs. In any case the choices here were also very limited. Not surprisingly, all presented the same guidelines, which – were the same as the WHO ones. The only important exception was that the country's name and emblem were on the cover page. Unbelievingly, I used to wonder why this exercise was deemed so necessary, that treatment initiation had to be deferred when the disease was so rampant. However, I presumed that the WHO must have had one important, uncertain, question in mind following their highly publicised treatment programme: would the pledges be honoured in full and in a timely manner? Would they satisfy the expectation that had been whipped up, or would they suffer condemnation for insensitively raising unrealistic expectations in the face of a truly human tragedy? While countries were kept busy, these questions would be blunted.

The prospects for a successful implementation of the UNAIDS 3 by 5 global initiatives did not look good. Right from the beginning, it did not look like an effective emergency relief operation. Ominously, the promised funds were slow in coming and fell grossly short of the pledged amounts. Many rich countries were put to shame by some poor ones who contributed more in relation to their income per capita. As a result the WHO could not conceivably meet the set targets. Meanwhile, the intended recipient countries were kept busy engrossed in writing national treatment guidelines. Those countries, including Uganda, that acted promptly and expeditiously found that by the time the national guidelines were really needed, they were already out of date. They had to do a second edition, which turned out - to be the same as the second edition of the WHO guidelines.

As the GAF kitty was only half empty, those concerned initially appeared to be paralysed to act on their own pledge to deliver treatment to the poor counties that were impatiently waiting for the promised reprieve. The big problem was the equity issue. To whom do you give the scarce money; whom do you leave out and on what basis? The GAF secretariat and WHO could, of course, not be seen to engage in any distribution arrangement that could in any way be construed as either inequitable or ineffectual. However, the options were problematic. If, for instance, the meagre funds were distributed equally among needy countries, it would have been far too small to have an impact in any country. There would be no success stories to talk about. Therefore, GAF and WHO appeared to absolve themselves of full responsibility. They placed instead the onus on the poor countries. It was up to them to write up their own national treatment proposals for a competitive award of the desperately-needed drugs. This had an additional advantage that some slow-responding donor countries could have extra time to honour their pledges and boost the fund. Of course, no such programme had ever existed before, and hence no experts existed in any country to quickly write up the grants application. Neither was there a ready expert panel to assess and impartially grade the applications. A team to work with the secretariat was scrambled to handle the matter, and once more consultants fanned out to help poor countries write up the lengthy applications. The proposals were to be judged and scored to decide who would win the award. Those whose proposals were unsuccessful, in reality meaning that they did not fit within the limits of available funds, had only themselves to blame. GAF management had to be seen to exercise both fairness and transparency, and the equity concerns appear to be addressed.

Although this exercise mirrored the well-established principles for awarding research or some special donor grants, I have never known this method to apply to a catastrophic emergency like a tsunami or AIDS. Was it morally and ethically acceptable that poor and distressed people should be taken to task, competing for life saving relief? Singing for one's dinner is perhaps excusable but having to sing for your life is a matter perhaps only the Hague international human rights court can judge. Is it determinable to choose between equally desperate people who can live and who can be let die on the basis of the grade of a written proposal? Is this any different from other kinds of discrimination? In such situation it only ensures the survival of the most competitive, leaving those who score lower to their fate.

The net effect of all this was that the money could not be quickly utilised to save lives, though somehow the programme boasted of having given out the first round of grants within three months. In reality, it had to wait for the bureaucratic process to take its course. The GAF and WHO were organisations constrained by red tape and so failed to respond to a humanitarian emergency while sitting on the desperately needed resources even if they were insufficient. As a result, some rich countries and organisations contemplated setting up their own AIDS relief programmes, hoping to deliver a more responsive emergency relief. In hindsight, this was not the kind of precedent that should have been set, because it undermined the WHO, which is widely relied on by poor developing countries as a guarantor of their health in a commercially-driven world. In truth WHO tries hard despite very difficult problems dealing with diverse countries with different bureaucratic problems and diverse interests. However, this does not entirely let WHO and UNAIDS off the hook, as their initial record in terms of success against AIDS was abysmal.

WHO and especially UNAIDS love slogans. They may be considered good for motivation or as goals to aspire to even if not eventually met. In fact before the 3 by 5 slogan, WHO had another slogan, which like the 3 by 5 strategy, also flopped. It was "Health for all by the year 2000". When the year 2000 came AIDS was the number one global health issue, and life-saving treatment was available, yet it was denied to the largest number of desperately ill people in history. One knows that these targets should not be taken literally but WHO should not make them so casually when they are obviously going to be far off target. They are a kind of indirect psychological torment (though unintended) to those desperately in need, whose hopes are raised only to be brutally let down. Admittedly, these were difficult times and issues for the WHO, and the answers were not necessarily straightforward, but the tough questions must be asked to protect against a repeat in future.

When GAF drugs finally arrived it was almost like an anti-climax. The drugs came in trickles called "rounds," creating a distribution dilemma for the few lucky countries that qualified for the money, or rather won the lottery. The first round of GAF drugs for Uganda was enough for just 3000 people out of an estimated 200,000 in immediate need. Politicians in Uganda took their cue from their WHO counterparts and also hit the publicity trail promising the battered population free drugs for all. These drugs were to be distributed equitably, transparently and efficiently, and then, of course, lengthy reports would be sent back to GAF and WHO on the positive impact. Reporting back detailing all steps of the programme and associated expenditure is vital to reassure the donors that their money is not being swallowed up in the notorious black hole of corruption generalised as endemic in Africa. Uganda - a country with over forty ethnic groups, five major religions, thirteen regions, sixty districts, and over 300 parliamentary constituencies - had the task of distributing the 3000 doses in a manner that took into account these factors on top of gender, age and special interest groups such as healthcare providers, teachers, orphans, pregnant women, and widows, to name some. Equitably! Yet the available drugs were enough for only 1.5% of those in a desperate battle for their life. No wonder one senior Ugandan politician affiliated to the Ministry of Health, who was awestruck and bemused by it all, found himself in a tight spot, when his colleagues cornered him to ask about the equity issue. Sloppily, he replied that the drugs would be distributed equally in all Ugandan parliamentary constituencies. He was not alone in this straight-jacket. Not many knew how to handle this awkward situation. The equity issue was taken so seriously that one hospital that was lucky to be allocated only 300 doses set out to demonstrate a transparent and equitable distribution of the drugs. A committee consisting of most district dignitaries and professional staff who had to leave their jobs to sit for days to select the 300 lucky ones from among the over 8,000 patients in need of therapy was set up. The majority who would inevitably miss out had heard about the donated free drugs. They can be forgiven if they assumed that they were victims of corruption, and blamed the healthcare providers or Ministry of Health officials for their misery.

As if the shortage within the GAF was not serious enough, the meeting in Abuja referred to earlier had looked beyond AIDS and tried to address the whole serious health crisis in Africa. They correctly decried the devastation caused by the two other African mass killer diseases, namely Malaria and Tuberculosis. Each of these two extensive and complex diseases deserved a separate fund-raising drive. The addition of these two diseases to draw from the same fund without corresponding increase in resources was sure to further diminish the effectiveness of the project for any of the three diseases. However, in the case of TB, which is linked closely with HIV, joint interventions were justifiable and inevitable, but required much more funding.

In the intervening period, the programme was off to a very slow bureaucratic start and the impression that many people got was that GAF and WHO were not competent. Therefore, as hinted earlier, some countries started planning their own AIDS relief initiatives, which they hoped would not be bogged down like GAF. Among other issues, this was one of the justifications for a separate President Bush Programme for AIDS Relief (PEPFAR) that was planned as a more rapid, less bureaucratic, more efficient and effective AIDS drugs access initiative. The best on earth!

Although the better funded and less bureaucratic PEPFAR was much more likely to succeed than the GAF, it was later to run into some pitfalls of its own.

Call to Washington

Late one evening in November of 2002, I was startled by a late evening call from Washington. Though I was still in my office in Kampala finishing off an urgent piece of work, it was far too late for official calls. It was from the National Institute of Health of the United States of America. On the line was none other than Anthony Fauci who said he wanted to talk to me rather urgently. Tony, as Fauci is popularly known around the globe, is the living guru of medicine. I knew very well that Tony just does not pick up a telephone and make late calls to the likes of me without a very compelling reason. I was thus jolted to attention as the details of his message unfolded. Instinctively, I sensed that there was something out of the ordinary in the offing, but little did I know that it had implications of life and death for millions of people around the world.

"I am calling to see if you could come to Washington." He just stated it simply, but I could detect a tone of urgency. Clearly, Tony was not merely exploring my availability for a possible visit. Unfortunately, this was just the wrong time for me to travel out of Uganda. I just could not, or so I thought, because my heart and thoughts were with a very dear friend who had just flown in especially for a reunion after about fifteen years. We had scheduled a holiday tour of the country, which just could not be interrupted.

"It is critically important," Tony added obviously sensing my hesitation. "We shall arrange everything for your travel and the visa - if you don't already have one, it will be handled for you."

"Well, I will need some time ..." I started, but he interjected cutting me short.

"I am afraid the matter is most urgent and we need you here almost immediately." He paused for a moment presumably to prepare me for the next part of his message. "Would you please start your journey tonight? I will arrange for a taxi to pick you up at Dulles Airport tomorrow and take you to your hotel." Tony concluded as if I had already accepted his invitation.

I faced a dilemma. How was I going to break the news about the abrupt change of plans to my visitor? In the circumstances, the visitor was very understanding, and nice about it all.

The next day I was on my way to Washington to attend to a very important matter that I knew absolutely nothing about. I went armed only with the trust that I had in Tony's word. Such is the power of the man! When I arrived at my hotel, I found a message redirecting me to another one on Pennsylvania Avenue. There was no explanation why it was deemed necessary to change, but I presumed that it was because the new one was closer to the venue of the meeting.

The first meeting was scheduled for mid-morning of the next day. The next morning I learned that the venue of the meeting was within the White House complex. I was joined in the hotel lobby by two familiar faces, Dr William Pape from Haiti, and Dr Paul Farmer from Harvard University, who also worked in Cange, a remote part of Haiti where he was involved in pioneer work on AIDS care and treatment; and one other expatriate American doctor working on a research project in Rwanda. On our way to the venue we stopped briefly at a café, as we still had some time before our meeting was due to start. While we sipped coffee, I got my very first idea of what it was all about. Paul and William already had the information that it was about AIDS treatment, and that the White House decision makers wanted information from the people in the field, especially the developing countries, to inform a new policy by the US government. Most of those we were to meet were Republican conservatives, not traditionally associated with the issues of developing countries, especially AIDS.

When the meeting got underway it was much more complicated than I had expected, and there were also much at stake. Obviously the special committee that we met had been debating the subject matter for quite some time. They had evidently gone over the contentious issues but did not appear to have come to a consensus, thus our summons. The committee consisted mainly of a Republican think tank, trying to work out US government policy in response to the global AIDS scourge with regard to treating the massive numbers of people who were dying a mainly preventable death. The background to the initiative could be traced back to President Bush's need to do something big on AIDS at the crucial time when America was preparing to go to war in Iraq. According to a public television special AIDS documentary, *Now*, presented by Brancaccio on November 4, 2005, which looked back at the events, President Bush had asked the government's experts "to hatch a plan." "And at the White House, momentum was building toward something big: a foreign aid plan that wouldn't just prevent AIDS, but for the first time, treat it. They devised one "which would blow the lid off any previous American efforts against global AIDS," Brancaccio reported in the programme.

As the US government had contributed a pittance to GAF, this was remarkable. But a series of events were responsible for this change of heart. First and foremost, there was the moral imperative. In Europe and the USA, some angry and compassionate citizens had for a long time been pressing their governments to do something for the poor of the world being devastated by AIDS. Secondly, America was preparing to go to war in Iraq, and it would not augur well for the USA to project to the world only an aggressive militaristic policy without a balancing empathetic and humanitarian element.

The highly respected Dr Anthony Fauci, the director of National Institute of Allergies and Infectious Diseases, was one of the top experts, who had pleaded for a strong and meaningful commitment of resources by the American government, enough to make a real difference to the suffering people especially in Africa. Tony was quoted on the same *Now* programme explaining the delicate situation that arose:

> And just as we were getting to the point of some decision making going on, they said. 'You know we can't just depend on you and a couple of your colleagues. We need to get some input from people who are actually in the field. Give us some models.'

It appears that some of the members had taken the then predominant view that committing funds to AIDS treatment in Africa was as good as just throwing it away. As explained in a previous chapter, this attitude was predominant because of the highly efficient lobby and system of misinformation orchestrated by business and ideological interests. As a result it was then widely believed that scaling up antiretroviral therapy was just too cumbersome for Africa. AIDS treatment was exaggeratingly described as high tech, requiring precision timing, state-of-the art laboratories, and highly trained experts. These "critical prerequisite needs" were described as unachievable in Africa. Many so-called experts made sure that this message was passed on to all influential politicians and especially the decision-makers among them. Worse still, some influential politicians were not even remotely interested in AIDS, especially in Africa. Some of them viewed it as just one of the numerous unsolvable problems in the developing world.

Among the most influential negative lobbies in Washington was the religious right, closely associated with the Republican Party. Their opposition could be traced back to the time when AIDS was first linked to homosexuality and sex in the early 1980s. The religious right included the influential Reverend Jerry Falwell, who in a televised sermon described AIDS as "God's punishment", and some extremists among them even welcomed AIDS as a just punishment for sinners who got what they rightly deserved for violating God's laws on sex. Naturally some among the religious right took exception to any public money being spent on AIDS. Instead some advocated repentance and sexual abstinence as the only acceptable intervention. They did not even absolve or forgive the numerous newborn babies that were dying of AIDS acquired from their mothers and refused to endorse any funding for the prevention of mother-to-child transmission. Presumably the little ones were visualised in their righteous lenses as guilty by association with the "sins" of their mothers. To the extremists, therefore, being born with AIDS would be construed as just an extension of God's punishment on the sinners. Yet incredibly at the same time, in an equally uncompromising stance, the same religious right extremists postured as crusaders to save the lives of other innocent babies. They were vehemently opposed to abortion under any circumstances in order to protect innocent lives, to such an extent that some were even prepared to kill for their strongly held belief. In fact a few actually did exactly that. Of course, the mainstream Republicans do not agree with the extremists but still, the Republican Party was at the very best of times always lukewarm about funding for AIDS. Some never wanted to hear anything about it, as Dr C. Everett Koop, American Surgeon General during the Reagan presidency was once rudely reminded. Dr Koop said in an interview with Brancacio on the Now programme:

Early on I was taken aside by the Assistant Secretary for Health, who was my immediate superior, and he said that in the scheme of things, I would not be required to do anything about AIDS. And.... it was enforced in a strange way. Whenever I appeared on, *Good Morning America,* or The Today Show, or something like that, there was always somebody from the public relations department who either preceded me or accompanied me and made it very clear to the anchor that I was not to discuss AIDS. And I was told, 'If you get a question, evade it.

The powerful North Carolina Republican Senator, Jesse Helms, was opposed to anything to do with AIDS because, as he once told the "New York Times," people only suffered from it due to their "deliberate, disgusting, revolting conduct." Many Republicans strongly opposed President Clinton's efforts to increase AIDS funding despite recognising the fact that it had broken the bounds of public health to become an international security issue. Clinton during his campaign for the presidency had promised massive funds to alleviate AIDS, in what he called a "modern day Manhattan project." Yet during the eight years of his administration spending on global AIDS rose from $125 million to a miserable $340 million, which in practical terms was as good as non-existent. Therefore with such varied and intransigent views on the emotive topic of AIDS, it was clear that our task in Washington was not going to be easy. I was to remain incredulous and combatant up to just hours before the actual announcement by President Bush during the 2003 State of the Union address.

My perception of the task at hand was first and foremost to make it abundantly clear that a state of catastrophic emergency existed in Africa as a direct result of AIDS. Many people in the USA did not appreciate the gravity of the matter. This critical issue was deliberately kept under wraps mainly for commercial interests and deviant views. We also had to impress upon the members that the sheer numbers dying an excruciatingly painful death constituted a moral imperative for the world's most powerful nation which had the power to stop the carnage but did not. I was absolutely convinced that unless these two points were explicit and appreciated well up front, no breakthrough could be expected. However, I had some reasons to be optimistic that if there was a good time to drive this point home in Washington, this was it.

In November 2002, the talk in Washington was almost exclusively focused on only one issue, and it was definitely not AIDS. All the electronic and print media, especially television news headlines, talk shows involving leading politicians and the public were all engrossed in the big debate about the looming Iraq war. The issue of whether there were weapons of mass destruction (WMD) about to be unleashed on the West or not was dividing the nation especially as it was increasingly becoming clear that the Bush administration was on the warpath. The souls and minds of the majority of the people in support of the war were crucial if the military campaign was to succeed. Therefore it would be prudent to counter the dissenting voices and all those who objected to their country increasingly being viewed as an uncaring aggressor of the weaker nations with a clear humanitarian agenda. There was probably no better way to show compassion than to reach out to the poor facing the world's worst catastrophe. After all, if "mass destruction" was what President Bush was out to stop, he would be spot on if he tackled the mother of all the world's mass destruction –AIDS.

This seemingly conducive atmosphere for the long-belated action on AIDS, however, did not necessarily mean that the deal was home and dry. There were other less controversial, but, of course, less deserving, humanitarian initiatives on the cards. The most predominant and influential opinion in Washington at the time advocated the same old token, cheap and easy-to-implement options, including the rather vague preventive programmes and the cheap Bactrim prophylaxis that were the favourite of most donors, and yet had little impact whatsoever on AIDS. The key to winning the battle of minds involved changing these deeply held views and refocusing attention on the real priorities that would make a difference. As we responded to the tough questions we explained that no AIDS intervention in Africa would make any meaningful impact or even be credible unless it addressed the critical issue of treatment. We dispelled the hackneyed excuses of infrastructure constraints, lack of human resources and logistics, not because they were not urgently needed, (in fact they were part of our recommendations), but because they were not legitimate excuses for denying help to the poor and the weak facing one of the most catastrophic disasters in history. We explained that the difficulties associated with the introduction of the complicated antiretroviral drugs could be overcome, and provided some models of Uganda and Haiti. We assured them that committing funds to AIDS treatment in Africa and other poor countries would save millions of lives and pay other dividends besides.

I explained that we had already developed the expertise to scale up ART in Uganda. My institution, the Joint Clinical Research Centre, had successfully extended AIDS treatment to a number of rural districts in Uganda. Using our model, I explained that we were ready to immediately scale up AIDS treatment and save lives if funds were made available. The experienced and no nonsense Paul Farmer was right there to reassure any doubting Thomases. "There are no special problems to stop treatment being administered in any poor set up, as demonstrated by our work in Haiti and other poor set ups," he explained. My other colleagues, based on their rich and practical experiences in poor countries, echoed the same message. The main constraint, we said in unison, was lack of drugs as they were just unaffordable. If the money could be found to purchase the drugs, lives would immediately begin to be saved as the other issues are addressed, we emphasized.

I left the meeting pleased and proud of our teamwork in advocating the urgent and critical need for help to stop the AIDS carnage in poor countries. I felt that we had inculcated a sense of urgency into the members to come up with a response to AIDS. However, conscious of the predominant conservative views of Republicans, I did not believe that it would translate into immediate action, and if it did, that it would be substantial. For this reason and others I will touch on later, I did not discuss my role with other people outside the inner circle, or talk about this important meeting or subsequent meetings until they were all over. Despite all our concerted efforts it transpired that there were still enough sceptics out there ready to stop our mission from being an outright fait accompli. Therefore, when I was again asked to go back to Washington, I was this time not taken by surprise. I assumed, and correctly so as I later found out, that the doubting Thomases were still not satisfied that massive AIDS treatment in Africa was either feasible or worth the required massive funding. To my consternation, on returning to Uganda, I had hardly unpacked my bags when the telephone rang.

"I hate to do this to you, Peter," the firm but apologetic voice of Tony was once more on the line. "I would be grateful if you could return to Washington immediately." After a brief pause he added, "I am sorry, and understand but it is important." I vividly recall an envious friend who irked me when he found out that having just returned from the USA, I was in the process of making a U-turn back. "You globe trotter," he reproached me. "I bet you keep a packed bag all the time!"

He obviously saw these as pleasure trips, and wished it were him enjoying the holiday bliss. This time round, however, I was rather fretful for two reasons. First of all I was rather tired and my mind was reeling trying to adjust to various time zones. Secondly I had just returned from Washington and therefore did not see what could be so desperately urgent that I had to go right back. Of course, I had no questions for Tony, as I was sure of his profound concern for the poor AIDS patients of the world and his personal dedication to do something about it. Though Tony had not been with us in the previous meeting, I knew his thoughts and mind were in our meeting room, because he too had been put through the mill. It was basically his recommendations that formed the basis of these intensive discussions. Indeed, in Tony, Africa has a hero. I do not personally know of any other American who did so much to get life saving therapy to Africa. If he, an American, felt so strongly then I had absolutely no excuse. It was back to the airport and off to Washington to be met by the freezing January weather.

This time however, every thing was different. The meetings were much more serene, and the new venue very high profile. It was in the inner White House. The meetings started early and ended late. All my earlier colleagues were nowhere to be seen. I was alone with the resourceful Tony and sometimes with the pleasant and brilliant Mark Dybul. Tony and I explained issues and answered questions related to

AIDS treatment in resource constrained countries and what it would cost to do it. The meetings involved a circle of senior Presidential advisors and some hard-working technocrats including the Presidential speechwriter. Hard work aside, my stay in the White House was quite momentous. There was Dick Cheney passing by in the corridor, humming a song and looking like an ordinary mortal. I was to be received though briefly by the great woman, Condoleezza Rice; and I met other dignitaries including the chief US budget officer to whom I had the impudence to give my business card which was snatched off his desk by his assistant. It was clear that we were putting together a document on AIDS funding, to which I was contributing some important details, and by the looks of it I could sense that it was vitally important, because every detail was being checked and crosschecked. The people I worked with were very economical with explanations. Release of information was on the "need to know" basis and often at the very last moment. Therefore, I had no idea at the time of the full impact that the document, which we were working on, would have in Africa until it was almost complete.

Monday evening, January 27, 2003, the eve of the State of the Union address, after a hard day's work fine tuning, and crosschecking the details, I was asked somewhat casually to dress in a business suit for the next day's work at the White House. This was a rather strange request because I was always dressed in a suit, and the Americans are not usually too fussy about dress. On my way back to the hotel, I passed by a department store and used my credit card to pick up a new suit. I still did not think much about the strange request until the following day which would rank among the most memorable of my life. When I arrived at the White House early the next morning it was obvious that some of the staff had been working most of the night. I could tell by the red eyes, the cups of coffee, the wrinkled suits and the signs of creeping fatigue. Tony was right there making sure that our part of the work was proceeding well. If any questions arose about any aspect of AIDS treatment in Africa I was at hand to answer. By the looks of it, Tony too cannot have had much sleep over the past week or so but he kept going regardless. Then at about 11.30 am I was for the first time told in plain English that we had $15 billion for AIDS in the bag and that the President was going to announce it that very evening. We had spent considerable time discussing the need for big amounts of money to tackle global AIDS, especially in Africa, in which the figure of $15 billion kept coming up. However, the possibility of the Republican administration raising the Democratic President Clinton's $350 million to $15 billion looked to be expecting too much! We had emphasized that if the runaway AIDS epidemic in Africa was to be seriously tackled, this was about the level of funding that would begin to make a difference, and only if it was protected from the notorious bureaucratic zigzagging.

By lunchtime on that memorable day of fast-moving events another surprise was sprung on me. I was told that I was invited to the State of the Union address as a special guest of the First Lady, Laura Bush! As if I had not had enough surprises in a single day, I was also invited to the pre-State of the Union reception in the official Lincoln Hall in the White House, where I would meet all kinds of dignitaries and other distinguished guests. Tony seemed quite elated, and I could for the first time discern an expression of satisfaction on his face. However, he must have been rather taken aback by my rather incongruous reaction. He could see that I was just too cool while great things were unfolding all around us under our very eyes. The truth of the matter was that I was numbed by it all. I just couldn't completely believe it had happened. To be sure, I still wanted to hear it from the horse's mouth. I knew of too many people helplessly dying of AIDS. I had seen too many promises of aid and relief turn to dust. I had attended too many meetings that planned action against AIDS, but simply did not materialise, and I had seen too many desperate people's hopes raised only to be rudely shattered. In very rare cases where anything had materialised it had always turned out to be too little, bogus, or at best just token. Was this one going to be different?

Certainly, there was something new and special about this particular initiative. We were for the very first time talking meaningful amounts of money, but was it going to end up on paper and in media announcements, like the UNAIDS access initiatives and the big

Pharma's accelerated access? Or was it going to be swallowed up by the notorious red tape whereby the donated money ends up right back with the donor without anything to show for where it was intended and desperately needed? This was the point I made over and over again. The money needed to reach those in need and not be used to run a bureaucracy. I had urged that AIDS funding should be treated like the emergency that it was, and therefore be dispatched urgently, unlike the GAF that seemed to be bogged down in formalities. The modus operandi itself could make it succeed or fail. Now that the much craved for relief finally looked closer, I found myself asking all these hard questions. The bottom line was that I would not count it done until I heard with my own ears the President of United States announcing it. In our long discussion it was always emphasized that, "The President of United States does not announce any programme already leaked to the public." Only the President could savour the glorious moment and receive the applause. In this case it was vitally important as he was also announcing a move towards the controversial Iraq war. The missile and the white dove were set to fly out together. It was like the classical stick and carrot scenario. However, even at that hour I had my fingers crossed. It was a tense moment for me. There was always the possibility that the President would announce something else.

Tony, kindly went out of his way make sure that I grasped the importance of the rapidly unfolding historical events. "Peter, you will be on worldwide television this evening," Tony said. "All cameras will be swinging to you! Peter, don't pick your nose …or make faces as this will be captured on tape and make news," he added jokingly. TV images were the last thing on my mind. The reverberating thought in my mind, as the Americans would put it, was just, *"Was it gonna happen?"* I meant the $15 billion.

All the specially invited guests had numbered seat tickets for the "Royal Box" and mine was number two. Number one belonged to Laura Bush. The reality of being a special guest of the First Lady of United States really hit me as we drove to Congress from the White House with police motorcycle outriders clearing the way, and then I was being ushered into my seat to await the arrival of Laura to take her seat next to me. I was struck by the fanatical clapping and standing ovations by Republicans at almost anything the President said, while the Democrats frowned at what they did not like and only clapped selectively on points coincidental with their own policies. However, when it came to AIDS, there was almost full unanimity as virtually everyone gave the President a standing ovation, as he said:

> Today on the continent of Africa nearly thirty million people have the AIDS virus, including three million children under the age fifteen. There are whole countries in Africa where more than one third of the adult population carries the infection. More than four million require immediate drug treatment. Yet, across that continent, only 50,000 AIDS victims - only 50,000 - are receiving the medicine they need. Many hospitals tell people, 'You've got AIDS, and we can't help you. Go home and die.' In an age of miraculous medicines, no person should have to hear those words."

Those words brought my antennae out, wondering with trepidation whether the deal was home and dry, but the speech continued,

> Tonight I propose the Emergency Plan for AIDS Relief, a work of mercy beyond all current international efforts to help the people of Africa. This comprehensive plan will prevent seven million new AIDS infections, treat at least two million people with life-extending drugs and provide humane care for millions of people suffering from AIDS and for children orphaned by AIDS. I ask the Congress to commit $15 billion over the next five years, including nearly $10 billion in new money, to turn the tide against AIDS in the most afflicted nations of Africa and the Caribbean. This nation can lead the world in sparing innocent people from a plague of nature.

These words sounded to me like melodious music!

I did not need to hear anymore. I was up in a flash clapping like a fanatical Republican, all my previous disbelief and anxiety allayed. This without any doubt was the brightest hour in my long years working without hope among the wretched of the world - the poor AIDS patients who were doomed to suffer and die an excruciating death simply because of their poverty. These words defined a turning point. No wonder, when I met the President after the speech, I was still so thrilled by the announcement that as we posed for the pictures, I just found I had inadvertently embraced his wife as the cameras snapped. It was just as well that the President was not a jealous husband. This crowned the day that was to change AIDS treatment and give so many people hope and life.

That is if it was to go all the way according to plan.

Hitting the Ground Running

When my centre, the JCRC, was awarded the President's Emergency Programme for AIDS Relief (PEPFAR) grant that resulted from President Bush's State of the Union address that I attended, to scale up ART in the rural areas in Uganda, we hit the ground running. We had been ready for over ten years, waiting just for an opportunity like this to materialise. However, when the offer was first made through USAID to JCRC my immediate reaction was to refuse it outright. I feared that the USAID highly bureaucratic system would spend time and money on setting up a bureaucracy instead of providing the urgently needed life-saving AIDS treatment. I knew of a number of donor supported projects that were not tailored to the local needs and agenda and ended up without anything to show for the funds. In fact, a number of them ended up as aid to the donor country itself as all the highly paid managers including the Chief of Party (COP), and most of the workers were expatriates. Often some of the experts lacked the relevant experience and were unfamiliar with local conditions. Some were selected on the basis of having written a college thesis on a vaguely related subject not always specific to the job at hand, or else on the basis of having spent a short time in a developing country. The COP and his team excel in writing elaborate reports to the donor. In fact, their success is measured in terms of the "quality" of reports they write, not always on what they actually achieve on the ground. Writing reports is a priority with most funded projects. In some cases the data and report writers outnumber the technical staff executing the actual project objectives. If there were a choice between a candidate who will do the job and achieve results and another one who could not necessarily do the job well but was able to make good reports, the latter would often be preferred. I detested being diverted from my critical work of patient care to be turned into a full time clerk. I made my position clear and suggested that they try another organisation instead, unless, of course, they were prepared to address my critical concerns.

Another concern on my mind was that some donors were not sensitive and supportive of locally developed best practices and initiatives. They just present a blueprint of their own ready for implementation. At the JCRC we had built our home-grown best practices which, against all the so-called insurmountable problems, had succeeded in introducing ART to Uganda and had saved a considerable number of lives without any foreign donor funds. In the process we built local expertise and capacity. I knew from experience that some funded donor projects had in the past destroyed all that had been achieved, leaving nothing to replace it when they left. Sometimes donor projects in Africa just ended often without warning and once the expatriates had gone home, the host countries were left once again to start from scratch. I, felt therefore, that it would be best for the JCRC to make it clear right from the beginning that we intended to do a serious job of saving lives based on the best practices that we had developed and successfully tested out. I sincerely believed, and with good reasons too, that our methodology was the most appropriate and most likely to succeed. I felt that our way would ensure continuity and sustainability when the donor project eventually ended or got fatigued. There were always many other organisations who would be pleased to accept the work under the donors' terms. My stand was rather surprising to the aid officials because many in poverty-stricken countries would have unquestioningly jumped at the mere mention of the offer.

However, I was later happy to change my mind and accept to work with USAID for several reasons. First, and most pleasantly, genuinely humanitarian officers represented the USAID. There were the affable Rob Cunane and the kind Amy Cunningham, who listened to my concerns and appreciated the importance of the issues that I raised. Not surprisingly both had in-depth knowledge about donor issues in developing countries and were therefore sympathetic to my strongly held points of view. They offered to discuss my concerns with their superiors and see whether they could be accommodated. They came back with a positive response and the two were to play an important role in quickly getting the life-saving treatment to thousands of Ugandans. Secondly, having fought so hard and for so long I was not about to let this unique opportunity pass by. Instead I would insist on getting assurances that the project was modelled on our own approach. Indeed I knew first hand, and more than many people, of the devastation of AIDS on our people. With PEPFAR funds I was sure that we would immediately build the capacity to alleviate the suffering of our people and save thousands of lives. I therefore had a moral obligation to accept the offer.

I was determined that our project would be different, although I knew that this could be difficult as many people of different backgrounds and ethical principles would be involved. However, I was determined to do all that was possible to avoid the pitfalls of most other donor projects, especially the bureaucratic impediments. When it was announced that we had been awarded the grant, we did not have to wait for it to clear the red tape that normally takes a long time. Instead, we immediately started our work of expanding treatment to the districts under the project acronym of TREAT, standing for Timetable for Regional Expansion of Antiretroviral Therapy. We caused raised eyebrows when we presented the receipts earlier than expected. In so doing, we had no apology to make because we had full accountability; and after all, the entire project was about addressing a catastrophic emergency. We only did it in the way in which emergencies should be addressed.

Immediately we started opening up ART satellite centres in all regions of the country prioritising areas where there were many patients in need. As we had a ready developed and proven methodology of establishing new centres that was to be known as "the network model" the expansion went well according to plan. The plan incorporated special approaches aimed at breaking the AIDS stigma. The opening ceremonies for new centres were always big celebratory occasions, that included marches and parades involving people living with AIDS, politicians, community based organisations, local leaders including religious leaders, and school children. The parades were led by brass bands and we staged impressive concerts. AIDS support groups performed plays and sang moving songs with AIDS preventive messages, alternating with speeches and information about AIDS prevention and treatment. This has since been adopted by other organisations as the best practice. I marched in all regions of the country as we opened more and more centres.

We ensured that the opening ceremonies involved as many prominent personalities in the country as possible to demonstrate that AIDS was the concern of all from the very poor to the pinnacle of society. It was a calculated strategy to break the stigma of AIDS which was the main constraint in seeking Voluntary Counselling and Testing (VCT) as well as AIDS care and treatment services. The marches showed everybody united against AIDS, and that it was not just the concern of infected individuals. It was also a great opportunity for Information, Education, Communication and Dialogue (IECD), and probably the only opportunity in each area that involved such a diversity of people all focused on care, treatment and prevention of AIDS.

The area woman Member of Parliament joined in the colourful opening ceremony in the eastern town of Mbale close to the Kenyan border. It coincided with the victory celebration for another popular local politician thus ensuring us a wider audience for us. In the ancient Kingdom of Bunyoro, in the main town of Hoima of western Uganda, bordering the Democratic Republic of Congo, the community was spellbound by a huge march that included the US ambassador, political and community leaders, schoolchildren, orphans, and community groups led by the Ugandan Army brass band. The big opening ceremony took place at the main sports stadium, where the Ugandan First Lady, Janet Museveni, was the guest of honour. In attendance was none other than Her Majesty, the Queen of Bunyoro, among many other prominent dignitaries. The mammoth crowd listened to the First Lady as she delivered her speech in which she emphasised the importance of strengthening AIDS prevention in the era of ART. I took the opportunity to describe the proper effective use of antiretroviral drugs and warned about the grave dangers of misuse ranging from toxicity and ineffectiveness to outright resistance. As was my usual theme, I advised that drugs must always be obtained from and used under the guidance and supervision of trained care providers only. I told the audience of my then famous three word formula vital for antiretroviral treatment success, namely: Compliance! Compliance! Compliance! Then, as was my practice at all rallies, I warned against complacency as the drugs were not an AIDS cure, and advocated continued vigilance in prevention since the drugs did not entirely stop transmission of the infection.

Further south, the Minister of Health personally presided over the opening of the Catholic Mission Hospital ART clinic at Nyakibale after a parade around the nearby dusty town of Rukungiri. Months later I was back in the area to open Ishaka Adventist Mission Hospital clinic where the Minister of Local Government presided, and proceeded to the launch of the Anglican Kisizi Missionary Hospital clinic, a hundred kilometres away where Bishop Muhima of North Kigezi was the main guest.

Other ART centres opened included Buhinga Hospital in the west, where the local Muslim leader led the opening prayer; Kabale in the south; Gulu and Lira in the north; and Jinja, Kakira, Iganga, Mukuju, and Soroti, in the east. In fact, we had at least one clinic in every province and were on course to open a clinic in each and every district where there was need.

Suddenly it looked like my marching days were rapidly coming to an end. Dizziness and an impending mighty fall seemed poised to bring it to a sudden stop. I was right behind the truck with music roaring from four huge loud speakers mounted on top, in the remote Ugandan eastern town of Ngora in Teso District, leading yet another march consisting of healthcare providers including nurses and doctors, school children, a women's group and people living with AIDS as villagers joined in at will greatly swelling the numbers. It was a hot sunny Saturday midmorning on February 26, 2005. The seven kilometre return march had started from Ngora Anglican Mission Hospital and was destined to take us through the once picturesque mission campus with a number of schools, chapels, and a church now surrounded by overgrown bougainvilleas, through the neighbouring settlements which were now a bat infested pale shadow of their former glory. We were to proceed on to the nearby small trading centre and back for the opening ceremony of our 26th Antiretroviral Treatment Centre. The tree lined potholed rough track necessitated a constant watch of one's steps to avoid tumbling into the numerous ditches, but in so doing I found that I could not properly coordinate my steps and balance. I felt myself heading for a big fall. But the problem did not seem to be solely due to the jagged terrain, as the ground level also seemed to swing high and swing low like the ancient Negro spiritual song says. If, for instance, the level appeared to be down I would adjust the next step accordingly only to hit the ground unexpectedly at a higher level with a thump. The next step, far from compensating for the previous error, would aim higher only to find that the ground had unexpectedly shifted down, making the stumbling walk much worse. The net effect of all this was more dizziness and confusion as the brain tried in vain to adjust to the incongruous signals.

The physician part of me sprang into action trying to analyse and diagnose the problem. Was it brain pathology, a blood circulatory disorder, a metabolic problem or just fatigue? Fatigue could be easily justified, as the previous two years had been very hectic, with the Joint Clinical Centre rapidly expanding ART access to many parts of Uganda. In fact, a treatment revolution was in progress. The marches were only part of a carefully designed strategy for the effective introduction of the new ART drugs to the districts. It used to be said that starting treatment in rural districts in Africa was impossible. Here we were doing the impossible on an almost fortnightly basis. We opened many new AIDS treatment centres with a big bang and became the talk of the towns and villages for a long time afterwards.

That fateful Saturday morning in Ngora, it looked to me like it was the very twilight of my marching days. We were just gearing up for greater parades ahead in other parts of the country. We planned to launch at least nine more treatment clinics in the following six months. Yet here I was being forced by seemingly failing health to quit the march. To me failure was not an option and I strong mindedly decided to carry on marching regardless. However, as the march gathered pace, the problem worsened. I worried that people would notice my predicament. How would anyone interpret the gait of a fellow who swayed, staggered, and stumbled? The hot weather was not helping, together with mounting anxiety. Sweat started pouring down my face misting my glasses. I swiftly removed them as I stretched out the other hand to offset an impending fall. Then, all of a sudden, my head cleared and I felt fine and stable! Energy and bounce returned to my steps as if it had all been merely a bad dream. I continued on the march with rather exaggerated military steps to correct whatever impression anyone might have gathered from seeing my frail, unsteady gait moments before.

After cleaning the sweat off the glasses, I put them back on, but, the problem was right back with a vengeance. The ground once more swayed, and dizziness and staggering resumed. All of a sudden I realised that it was my new bifocal lenses playing tricks on me. It was worsened by the rough terrain that required me to glance frequently up and down to avoid hitting something, thus registering different focal points in quick succession. I felt an overwhelming sense of relief that it was none of the possible imaginary calamities that I had begun to fear were responsible. My glasses safely in my pocket I was already looking forward to future marches.

Epilogue

The Next Inferno

Harrowing may not adequately describe the AIDS carnage in Sub – Saharan Africa. The massacre still continues though at a slightly lower level than during the bleak decade of 1995 to 2005. Yet unbelievably, for the whole bloody decade highly effective medicines that could have saved millions existed, and technology existed to mass produce them for all easily.

In history, this was not an isolated incident, except perhaps for the vastness of the causalities, and the viciousness of the disease. Otherwise, many episodes in history testify to numerous other raw deals for the world's poorest continent. Whenever Africa, dubbed the Dark Continent, is faced with catastrophe the world's compassion almost always falls short. The response, if any, trickles in slow motion, and the help that materialises, if at all, is almost always too little or too late. Sometimes it has been left to rock bands to stage concerts to help Africans hit by devastating drought or flooding, often attributed to greenhouse gases generated mainly in other continents. Even when some charitable initiatives were staged, Africans who sought to participate in the fund raising drive got a raw deal. In one such event, African artistes were excluded from the main venue on the pretext that no one really knew them and they would therefore not attract donors. They were sent to perform in an obscure venue where hardly anyone saw them, because all attention was focused on the main event. Of course, it was true that the artistes were unknown, and I like to believe that the motive for relegating them to this venue was in good faith, but that was precisely the point. This could have been the time - a unique opportunity for them to get known. No one said they were not talented.

Even by the usual standards of mean treatment, the pitilessness in the case of AIDS devastation was excessive. Africa cried her heart out for help to alleviate the carnage of AIDS – which posed the biggest threat in her history because it threatened a massive genocide. The continent was faced with a "towering inferno" - but her cries and pleas fell on very deaf ears. It is not that the world owes Africa a living, but all humanity is at least entitled to basic humanitarian emergency relief when calamity strikes. This is the very basic definition of humanity. Yet, shamefully, in the case of the mother of all disasters, AIDS, international relief was conspicuous by its denial, which resulted in severe suffering and a disastrous loss of lives.

The little that had been achieved by the 2005, in terms of access to AIDS drugs for the poor countries, only started in 2003, two decades after AIDS was discovered and almost a decade after highly effective drugs were discovered. The relief came after a long drawn-out hard fight involving forces of compassion, human right's activists, lawyers, shocked healthcare providers, the long-suffering patients and their families and a rare stroke of luck. Yet the outcome, measured in terms of what remains to be achieved, still puts mankind to shame.

It is appalling that by 2005, life-saving drugs were still inaccessible to over 70 percent of those desperately fighting for their very lives. Therefore, the work that still lies ahead makes what has been achieved look petty in comparison. To succeed, the current level of donations and other efforts need to be at least trebled if they are to stand any chance of gaining the upper hand in the still unfolding crisis. One of the main hitches remains the formidable roadblock enacted by drugs patent holders. The new worrying aspect of it is the imposition of an international requirement that all drugs known after the cut-off date of 1996 be given special protection so that the companies who supposedly invested "huge amounts of money" could get a return on their investment. The exception so far is powerful Brazil which was granted an extra year of grace to make the necessary arrangements. This means that the rules addressing today's AIDS treatment issues were backdated by ten years! If this appears sadly retrogressive, that is perhaps what it may be. Brazil's ordeal in 2005 during her skirmish, euphemistically dubbed "negotiations," with pharmaceutical companies sends chills down the spines of the poor AIDS ridden countries which will almost inevitably fare much worse. Brazil is a very wealthy country when compared to almost all African countries, with the possible exception of South Africa. It has a highly developed ART access programme, but it has an easier job because it has a much smaller AIDS burden than Sub-Saharan African countries.

Under the terms of the 1996 TRIPS deadline scheme, AIDS drugs known before 1996 may continue to be produced by generic manufacturers, but not those known after that time. What is so crucial about this timing? This again, as always, has to do with business. There is no longer any strong incentive to defend the monopoly on AIDS drugs known before 1996 because these drugs are now second class in the West, and the patents mandatory period is due to expire for some. Advances in research have produced a newer generation of AIDS drugs that are safer and more effective than those known before 1996, downgrading the old generation of AIDS drugs to the almost exclusive use of poor countries. As they are also relatively easy to manufacture, a growing list of countries is either manufacturing the drugs or are preparing to do so. Also, the generic manufacturers have successfully formulated these same drugs into fixed dose combinations. The combined formulation drugs comprise two or three drugs previously patented by different companies, which had been marketed and priced independently and thus were very expensive.

The AIDS drugs increasingly out of favour in the West include Stavudine a drug that is still commonly used in Africa. Others being used less commonly in the rich countries include Zidovudine, and to some extent Nevirapine. These drugs have several aspects in common: besides being no longer the first choice drugs in rich countries they are no longer the money-spinners they used to be. Stavudine especially is associated with serious side effects, which are just unacceptable in the West because of the availability of the much safer alternatives. Yet these drugs, albeit second-class in rich countries, are still the main lifeline for AIDS patients in poor countries simply because they are cheaper and the ones that available donor money can buy in bulk. To the poor, such drugs were still acceptable since they had no access to the modern, less toxic alternatives and yet without them the only other alternative was death. However, those who donate these kinds of drugs to the poor and yet could afford the safer and more effective alternative therapy should bear in mind the full for reality of their actions. They are only swapping one kind of agony with another. The difference is just the severity between the two degrees of suffering.

Another hovering danger that Africa should brace for is widespread AIDS drugs resistance. By and large, drugs resistance is to some extent almost inevitable. All that can be done about it is to delay it for as long as possible by slowing down the multiplication rate of the virus. Resistance, explained in easy terms, results from errors in the succession of the building micro blocks (amino acids) of the virus otherwise known as mutations, which occur during the process of multiplication, or copying itself. Some resultant changes may confer drug resistant properties to the new configuration virus that then acquires the ability to escape the effect of the drugs. As copying mistakes occur only during multiplication, the more the multiplication the more chances of mutations. In addition, selection for resistance against a specific drug is most likely if the virus is able to multiply in the presence of the drug, for instance when the drug is sub-optimal or only partly effective. In such a situation, the resistant mutants will be selected for multiplication since they can escape the effect of the current drug. In actual fact all micro-organisms undergo mutations. Mutations are the mothers of resistance to drugs. The fathers are multiplications. In the case of poorly treated HIV infection the multiplications take place at high-speed making copying mistakes very common. Without treatment, billions of viruses multiply in a single patient every day. The only way to minimise mutation is to slow down the multiplication of the virus. And this is exactly what ARVs do, provided they are used properly and the virus is not resistant. Unfortunately, the current drugs do not stop the multiplication of the virus completely. As long as there is multiplication taking place some degree of mutation is inevitable. To ensure that mutation, and therefore resistance, is kept at bay for as long as possible one has to ensure optimal usage of the drugs which ensure the lowest possible viral copies. The two cardinal rules for the best possible use of AIDS drugs in any treatment programme are to make absolutely sure that there is adherence, supported by uninterrupted drugs supplies, competent medical supervision, and that timely action is taken to address any resistance as soon as possible when it occurs so that it does not become more complex and go on to become resistant to other possible substitute drugs.

However, there are special factors that make AIDS resistance in the poor countries of Africa especially ominous. First of all, the epidemic was left to reach such a calamitous stage engulfing huge numbers of people, currently estimated at over thirty-five million. The belated and half-hearted action that was later taken was far too little and too late. It was initially just a drop in the ocean. The majority of people who were lucky to access the drugs were already very sick, making it more likely for the treatment to fail. Part of the definition of "failure of AIDS treatment" is that resistance has developed. Therefore, starting treatment late augments resistance to drugs. There were also too few drugs, meaning that the vast majority of people in desperate need of them were not able to access them. It was a nightmare for healthcare providers with insufficient drugs who were forced into the agonising position of having to make a choice that only God should make: to choose among desperately ill patients whom to give the lifesaving drugs to and whom to deny them. In almost all drugs-donor programmes this unpleasant issue was always left to the recipient countries to sort out. However, there was always a condition requiring all recipients of donated drugs to make absolutely sure that drugs were equitably distributed, despite the grossly deficient amounts. In some instances, it was like casting a lot to determine who lives or dies. The lucky few - if that is what you would call those selected to access the few drugs available - would be faced with the plight of seeing other family members suffering from the same disease go without. I saw many in such a situation. They included one tearful woman who once turned up in my clinic, threw the one month's supply of antiretroviral drugs she had obtained from a charity clinic on my table, and started to walk out. I implored her to at least explain what it was all about. She explained that a month earlier she had gone to an AIDS clinic with her sick husband and daughter when she heard that there were free AIDS drugs available there. Though all three were assessed to require therapy, all they could accommodate was treatment for just her alone.

To the clinic's credit, she was well counselled about adherence and warned against sharing out the drugs.

"I just can't take these drugs doctor," she said sobbing. "Taking the drugs while my family dies makes me feel like a wicked witch!" As I shifted uneasily in my chair trying to find something reasonable to say to her, she had something more to add. "I have been back to the clinic and begged them to put my daughter on the treatment instead of me, but they said they did not have any children's drugs formulation." I could see that getting rid of the problematic drugs seemed to have lifted the burden of guilt off her shoulder, as she was getting more and more composed with time.

"What do you want me to do with the drugs?" I asked her.

"Please give them to some other patient who can use them, because I don't want them to go to waste when they can help someone out of this curse." Then she added resignedly but with apparent relief, "As for me I will die with my family."

I was caught up in the same kind of sad situation when two kind American women were touched by the plight of the two AIDS infected kids Molly and Samantha, filmed in the compound of a sister AIDS clinic in Kampala by CBS and aired in a *Sixty Minutes* documentary programme in the USA, under the title "Paying the Price." The programme featured the two-orphaned children who had struck a friendship during their frequent clinic visits and always had a great time playing together within the clinic's compound. However, one of them was ailing by the day as AIDS progressed. The other orphan was doing well because she was lucky to have a rich foster family able to afford the highly expensive antiretroviral therapy for her. The poor kid explained her fate in a sort of detached way while her friend looked on sorrowfully,

> "My friend will live because she has the drugs, and I will die because I don't"

The programme gave my address at the end of the chilling documentary, and the next day I was bombarded with emails of shocked and angry viewers. One irate viewer wrote, "You stupid and disgusting people, don't you know it is against the law to deny children treatment?" This person did not know that it was the law of the jungle that ruled in the world of hard-nosed drugs business interests. It is called survival of the richest. However, he was not the only one so ignorant of the real world order. There was yet another email also expressing shock, "We were told that AIDS was no longer a problem. How come you have this pathetic situation in your country?" All that the majority of the people in the West ever get to hear about AIDS and the pharmaceutical companies are the "very generous donations" and "huge cost reductions" frequently announced in a flurry of publicity extravaganza.

Pleasantly, there was a silver lining to this sad documentary. Some compassionate individuals sent donations to cater for the second child's treatment and happily the poor orphan did not have to talk in terms of death any more.

Two kind American women of modest means, who also watched the documentary, responded by combining their pension allowances and offered to support treatment for one orphan in our clinic. That was all they could afford. There were, of course, many orphans in the clinic and I just offered it to the first one in need of the life-saving treatment who came to the clinic soon after it became available. For the others who came that day I did what I had always done, which was to treat the opportunistic infections and offer them painkillers to alleviate their suffering. Soon after initiating the lucky child on treatment I travelled on official duty and when I returned a fortnight later, I was stunned by a big bill from our finance department that I was not aware of. It transpired that the foster mother of the lucky orphan had returned to the clinic with another orphaned boy with AIDS and lied to the staff that I had offered treatment sponsorship to him as well. I immediately sent for the mischievous woman, for a tongue-lashing. I planned to tell her of the many orphans we had in the clinic, and how lucky she was to find a sponsor for one of her orphans, how she had abused her privilege and so forth. However, when the obviously embarrassed poor woman turned up the next day with the hapless orphan in tow, aware that she was in for the high jump, I was just tongue-tied with shame. "Thanks for doing what you did for this child," I mumbled to her as her anxiety was replaced by puzzlement. "I will find some way to maintain his therapy," I concluded as she sighed with relief that she had gotten off so lightly.

The truth of the matter was that I had absolutely no idea of where I would get the money for the orphan's treatment. But what else could the poor woman have done? She could handle the situation when both her orphaned children were not getting therapy, but having to nurse one child to health and another one to his death was just insufferable! She was forced to lie for the child and felt so awful in the process. In turn she made me feel awful for blaming her for "being human."

With regard to the woman that returned the drugs, I could understand her plight. How many would take the drug to save their own skin, leaving a loved one to die, without suffering agonising guilt or at least considerable anxiety? This predicament was a widespread reality and left many desperate people with no alternative but to engage in acts that lead directly to the rapid development of resistance. These included sharing out drugs, taking drugs irregularly, using under dosages, getting alternative drugs, often fakes, from quacks, and/or self-medication. This is the direct consequence of giving out too few drugs for a killer disease. The sensible alternative to protect against this dilemma, as I have always advocated, is to provide the vital drugs at an affordable price which the relatively well-to-do can afford; and then prioritise the poor to access free ones universally.

Under prevailing circumstances early resistance is guaranteed unless there is a change of approach and direction. Our very preliminary research has confirmed what we have always feared: that the interruption of drug treatment due to unaffordable drugs is likely to drive resistance in poor countries. Therefore, it may be said that unaffordable prices contribute towards development of resistance in poor countries. So the lesson for all world AIDS relief programmes, including GAF, the World Bank and PEPFAR, is to aspire to provide truly equitable and universal access to AIDS drugs. Otherwise the poor countries need to immediately tighten their belts because massive drugs resistance is approaching fast unless strong action is taken right now.

This is not a vote of "no confidence" in the current drugs donations programmes. It is just a call for a more robust and effective programme that ensures, among other things, that drugs are delivered in a timely manner, side by side with a strong preventive initiative, so that we increase the chance of stopping the horrific epidemic in its tracks.

However, it is not only the prospect of resistance that is especially frightening. It is what lies ahead of resistance that is staggeringly distressing. Yonder stands a concrete roadblock unless it is opened. Almost all the drugs available to deal with the AIDS virus resistant to the first line drugs were discovered after 1996. The twenty years mandatory monopoly period guaranteed by patents laws will only start to expire after 2016. Before that time, all countries will register increasing cases of drugs resistance to first line drugs. The waters have been tested by Brazil because there are already a large number of patients in need of second line drugs. To negotiate access Brazil threatened to break the patents laws and was threatened with sanctions. When Africa's turn comes it will be yet a new round of struggle for access to drugs of such magnitude that the first round will look like child's play. If the lessons of the first round serve us right, any concessions will come too late. This would ensure that the second line drugs fail quicker, leaving a massive number of patients in need of third and salvage therapy. Then, God forbid, because a new super strain of the virus may have emerged by that time – Apocalypse?

Yet all this is not inevitable. New and still emerging diseases over the last quarter century have sounded a stern warning to the world. The era of global infectious diseases is upon us. We need to establish best practices to help us fight other epidemics and pandemics yet to emerge and not be caught unawares again. We have seen Hantavirus in the American West, Brazilian purpuric fever and West Nile virus (first described in north-western Uganda) breaking out in the USA. I have witnessed frightened passengers on airlines wearing masks for fear of contracting SARS, which first broke out in the East and spread to many parts of the world before it was controlled. More recently, there has been an outbreak of the bird flu virus that is being spread rapidly across Asia by migrating birds and is making its way across the

African continent. It is just a matter of time before some such disease breaks into a worldwide epidemic. There have also been outbreaks of the horrifying lethal hemorrhagic fevers like Ebola in central Africa; others too that are equally devastating such as the Lassa fever and the Marburg virus, an ape virus that emerged from the Democratic Republic of Congo and killed people in Germany. Then, still with us, is the current nightmare; the great AIDS pandemic that has killed and continues to kill millions of the poor and marginalised people of the world. AIDS is massacring people while the world has the treatment, and the means to stop it. This knowledge and the power to stop the scourge have been selectively used and very successfully so for the rich. With a possible super strain on the way the West may not be spared since AIDS needs no visa.

No one can be absolutely safe irrespective of geography or socio-economic status, especially as diseases now travel across continents, by ocean currents, aircraft, birds, animals, humans and other means, not excluding bio-terrorism. While the current horrific pandemic remains unresolved, no one knows how serious the next pandemics will be. However, everyone can be absolutely sure that as has been tragically demonstrated by the AIDS debacle, the current drug patents TRIPS and WTO laws do not give, humanity, especially the poor, a good fighting chance of escaping with their lives. Yet the needed rectification of these laws is vigorously opposed in order to protect insatiable business interests. Those who continue to plead that profits are essential to ensure that new drugs are innovated for humanity are not always right because there is evidence to show that the contrary is true. Under the current regime of profit-driven pharmaceutical industries, drugs for rampaging killer diseases like Sleeping Sickness are not being developed simply because they are not profitable. In fact, current AIDS drugs would not have been developed with as much sense of urgency (if at all) if the disease had been confined to Africa. No one I know has ever claimed that the AIDS drugs were developed for the poor who were in most desperate need. On the contrary, they were denied to the poor for so long because they could not pay the price. The very first meaningful AIDS drugs access programme for Africa became possible only when the US paid 15 billion dollars for the lifesaving drugs to begin to be released to the poor. However, this is neither a comprehensive nor a long term solution. This is due to the fact that the donation is not enough to provide therapy to all in need, and no firm commitment has been made for long term support as AIDS is a life-time disease.

In all fairness we need to appreciate that WHO and UNAIDS tried their best to help and I know many individual staff who did a wonderful job. Many of them were no less alarmed about the whole sorry saga than I was. In fact, some of them frequently went out of their way to advise and assist my struggle to increase access to AIDS drugs. WHO and UNAIDS are just a reflection of the member states and cannot do much more than the member states mandate them to do. Countless times I saw them pick up the pieces and try to alleviate a desperate situation, but not always succeeding in making a meaningful impact on the enormous problem. Inevitably as the bodies directly responsible for control of the epidemic at international level they faced severe criticism. They needed the commitment of the United Nations, especially the rich and influential members, to achieve anything for the suffering poor. As the GAF was a G8 and UN initiative, the representative bodies that determine what ticks on Earth, they also take some responsibility for the failure to address the global AIDS pandemic.

However, this is not also to say that both UNAIDS and WHO do not have room for improvement. Their overwhelming tendency to prematurely count their eggs before they are hatched, (e.g. "health for all by the year 2000"), announcements of successes when none is in sight (e.g. "UNAIDS Access Initiative"), building mountains out of mole hills or just hastily making unachievable promises, (e.g. "3 by 5") and dillydallying with the big business when they had nothing to offer, (e.g. "Accelerated Access Initiative") were the undoing in their handling of the AIDS pandemic. I think they would have done better by more intense lobbying of the powerful G8 and UN and by making it repeatedly and abundantly clear that this was the most serious human disaster facing the world that demanded visionary leadership, human rights and compassion. They should have mobilised all the AIDS devastated countries and together pressed the UN, insisting that AIDS be put at the top of the world's agenda. They should also have made it clear to the pharmaceutical companies that they would not accept any dubious programmes, and insisted on a more meaningful partnership which would make critical life-saving drugs truly accessible to all in need. Above all, they should have acted like they were dealing with a tsunami, although, in fact, the devastation of AIDS was worse in all aspects except that it was a slow killer. At the very least, they should have, over the course of ten years since HAART was discovered, devised new ways of ensuring universal ART access. However, there is still room for redemption, as some good can still be salvaged, despite the scores of millions of lives already lost, because AIDS is still rampant and there is still no end in sight. The flawed world order that allows such devastation to happen is still in place doing business as usual. A Moses to lead the world out of this wilderness has yet to emerge. Where is this Moses?

The most important lesson learnt so far is that our current world order is poorly prepared to protect us from the catastrophe that the next pandemics will bring, let alone see this one off. Some people have compared the world to a global village, but to me it looks very much like an estate instead. It is like an estate that is endowed with hills and valleys. The masters of this estate are not kind to the men, women and children living and working on it. The great masters, the "haves", are comfortably ensconced on the relatively disease-free hills while the muddling "have-nots' are swarming in the disease-ridden flooded valleys with no hope of climbing the slippery cliffs to escape. When they look up they see only bridges connecting the bountiful hills. However, these bridges provide only false security for those enjoying the bliss of the hills because the foundations and supports are built in the valleys. The supports need regular reinforcement by the people in the valley. If the disease weakens them and the heavy rains come with floods, the bridge will be washed away and the comfortable houses in the hills will come tumbling down.

Therefore, there is urgent need to drain the flooded valleys and terrace the hills, so that people can move up and down in peace, health and security, and so turn the hostile estate into a pleasant, compassionate and caring global village.

Laws that deny or delay access to life-saving and emergency drugs should be urgently addressed on the humanitarian principle of lives above profits, but without hurting the businesses. Innovation in the crucial area of human survival should not be entirely dependent on money-making and big business, but should primarily aim at the alleviation of all human suffering and saving lives as a basic minimum. This does not contradict fair trade. Business success and humanism are not incompatible It is just a big lie to suggest that humanity is too dim to find ways of rewarding innovation and discovery other than by holding the very weakest of our society at ransom. It is also untrue that the only way businesses can thrive is by cutthroat pursuit of profits under powerful and insensitive protective laws, irrespective of the misery caused and the trail of blood in their wake. Lessons learns from the AIDS disaster should help the world find a way of incorporating justice and human rights in business. It is glaringly clear that the ills of the present system need to be fixed.

Donations per se are not substitutes or a permanent solution to a life-long disease. Most of the issues that lay in the background to the massive AIDS deaths are well known, as are most of the solutions. It remains the world's collective responsibility and cardinal duty to always urgently aid humanity in times of disaster. The world must enact and operate under truly humanitarian international laws that unambiguously, equitably, and justly protect the lives of the weak in society. Otherwise, the fire next time may engulf our global village in a towering inferno.

References

Slim disease: a new disease in Uganda and its association with HTLV-III infection.
Serwadda D, Mugerwa RD, Sewankambo NK, Lwegaba A, Carswell JW,
Kirya GB, Bayley AC, Downing RG, Tedder RS, Clayden SA, et al.
Lancet. 1985 Oct 19;2(8460):849-52.

A new disease has recently been recognised in rural Uganda. Because
the major symptoms are weight loss and diarrhoea, it is known locally
as slim disease. It is strongly associated with HTLV-III infection
[Later to be known as HIV], (63 out of 71 patients) and affects females
nearly as frequently as males. The clinical features are similar to those
of enteropathic acquired immunodeficiency syndrome as seen in
neighbouring Zaire. However, the syndrome is rarely associated with
Kaposi's Sarcoma (KS), although KS is endemic in this area of Uganda.
Slim disease occurs predominantly in the heterosexually promiscuous
population and there is no clear evidence to implicate other possible
means of transmission, such as by insect vectors or re-used injection
needles. The site and timing of the first reported cases suggest that
the disease arose in Tanzania

Prevalence of HIV in East African lorry drivers. Carswell J,W et al,   AIDS 3(11)
759-761

The Dungeons of Nakasero by Wod Okello Lawoko, published by the author,
printed by Fortahares Bokmaskin, Stockholm March 2005.

*Truck drivers, middlemen and commercial sex workers: AIDS and the mediation of
sex in south western Uganda.* M. Gysels, R.Pool and K.Bwanika: AIDS care
(2001) VOL 13. No 3 pages 373-385

*Man who takes pride in Wife Inheritance: Scholars won't agree on the role of the
practice in the spread of HIV.* By Oscar Obonyo, Sunday Nation newspaper
(Kenya), Jan 15, 2006 Special Reports. Page 14

Thirty Tons of Soil: Nanyonga's Divine Panacea, By David Blumenkrantz
(November 1989).

People are dreaming if they believe that Nanyonga's soil will solve
their problems. It is true that there are natural remedies that help
any infections. Quinine from the bark of the cinchona tree can cure
malaria, and various herbs can help heal wounds and kill infections.

There is even a type of soil kaolin, a chalky clay which helps bind the stomach when people are suffering from diarrhoea. But there has never been any drug that can cure all diseases. What a wonderful thing that would be. (Editorial, *The New Vision*, November 11, 1989 quoted by David Blumenkrantz)

Zairean AIDS Researcher Remains the Centre of Controversy, Michael Roddy, Reuters 16 November 1998

A Zairean doctor who announced last year that he had discovered an effective, non-toxic cure for AIDS, recently announced a new and improved version of the drug. Dr. Lurhuma Zirmwabagabo last year reported the discovery of MM-1--named for Zairean President Mobutu Sese Seko and Egyptian President Hosni Mubarak--and this year said he and Egyptian colleague Dr. Ahmed Shafik had come up with MM-2. The doctors have yet to publish information about the drug, subject it to independent testing, or divulge what it is. The kindest word any other researcher has to say about MM-2 is that it should be independently tested. Shafik was recently banned from practicing in Egypt for six months.

Drugs Companies sue South African Government over generics, British Medical Journal, 24 February 2001, 322:447.

In Kenya HIV/AIDS has affected many families with some 2.2 currently infected with economic losses of as high as Kenya shillings 210 million or US$ 2.8 million daily. Statement by Hon. C.B.Okemo, Kenya's Minister for Finance on the occasion of Health and Finance Ministers meeting on mobilisation of resources for an expanded response to HIV/AIDS in Eastern, Central and Southern Africa. Held Safari Park Hotel, Nairobi 10th Aug 2000.

Children on the brink 2002: A joint report on orphan estimates and programme strategies. The Synergy Project, UNAIDS, UNICEF and USAID (2002). http//data.unaids.org/Global-Reports/Bangkok,2004/UNAIDS_Bangkok_Press/childrenonbrink2004.en.pdf

It used to be said that in Africa, there was no such thing as an orphan. This was because in many African communities, children who had lost their parents were traditionally taken in by members of their extended families, most often an aunt or an uncle. Today, however, the devastating impact of HIV/AIDS on the adult population of Africa has resulted in large numbers of orphans and far fewer aunts and uncles to take them into care. (Quotation from the Firelight Foundation on Children and AIDS: The crisis.)

The UNAIDS Pharmaceutical Industry initiative, Health Gap Coalition position Paper: "Questioning the UNAIDS/Pharmaceutical Industry Initiative: Seven months and counting ..." Presented at the UNAIDS PCB in Rio 13 December 2005. http/www.globaltreatment.access.org/content/press_release/2000

UNAIDS PRESS RELEASE, Geneva, 11 May 2000.

NEW PUBLIC/PRIVATE SECTOR EFFORT INITIATED TO ACCELERATE ACCESS TO HIV/AIDS CARE AND TREATMENT IN DEVELOPING COUNTRIES,

The Joint United Nations Programme on HIV/AIDS (UNAIDS) announced today that a new dialogue has begun between five pharmaceutical companies and United Nations organisations to explore ways to accelerate and improve the provision of HIV/AIDS-related care and treatment in developing countries.

The pharmaceutical companies involved - Boehringer Ingelheim, Bristol-Myers Squibb, Glaxo Wellcome, Merck & Co., Inc., and F. Hoffmann-La Roche - have indicated their willingness to work with other stakeholders to find ways to broaden access to care and treatment, while ensuring rational, affordable, safe and effective use of drugs for HIV/AIDS related illnesses. The companies are offering, individually, to improve significantly access to, and availability of, a range of medicines.

Pills profits Protests: A chronicle of the Global AIDS movement Documentary produced and directed by Anne - Christine d'Adesky, Shanti Avigan, and Ann Rossetti.

Today is the day when we say to the nations of the world, "Enough! Enough!" 21 million dead from AIDS is enough. 36 million people around the world infected with the HIV virus is enough. This coming week, the United Nations first ever General Assembly Special Session on HIV/AIDS will submit their resolution on their response to the global AIDS plague. Before they do, they will hear the demands of their citizenry. We affirm the demands of people living with HIV/AIDS in the global south for access to care, treatment and support. (AMANDA LUGG quoted in the documentary.

www.outcast-films.com/films/ppp/index.html

Congo Brazzaville Health data, Accessed 16 February 2000,
    http:data.unaids.org/publications/fact-sheet 01/Congo

Nevirapine donation Accessed 16 Jan 2006:

http:// www.boehringer -ingelheim.ca/news release/2003/2003-11-27.asp

BI donation, Accessed 16 Jan 2006,
    http://www.actupny.org/reports/durban-boehringer.html

Jonathan M. Fishbein, M.D., Accessed 20 February 2006. http://www.
    honestdoctor.org,

Nevirapine misinformation: will it kill? AIDS Treatment News, Nov-Dec, 2004 by
    John S. James. Accessed 20 February2006.
    http://www.findarticles.com/p/articles/mi_m0HSW/is_407-408/ai_
    n9485138/pg_2

ANC Accuses US of 'Conspiracy' in Nevirapine Trials Dec 20, 2004...pigs" and
    "enter[ing] into a conspiracy" with a German pharmaceutical manufacturer
    to conceal potential adverse effects of the antiretroviral drug Nevirapine.
    ... - *Medical News Today.*

Don't confuse Nevirapine users: TAC Dec 15, 2004

> "The safety of single-dose Nevirapine is not in question, the Treatment
> Action Campaign re-iterated today, following comments by the
> department of health. ... " *SABC News.*

Nevirapine notes and references from the press:

> Allegations of "airbrushed and cooked damning clinical data
> from a large experimental trial in Uganda that tested a drug called
> Nevirapine". *New York Press.*

> Articles about AIDS drug trial prompt outrage in Africa Fraud ...
> - Articles by the Associated Press last week detailing allegations of
> incompetence and fraud in clinical trials of the drug, Nevirapine, have
> been interpreted. *San Francisco Chronicle,* Dec 21, 2004

> Allegations Raise Fears of Backlash Against AIDS Prevention - ...
> series last week that has reignited debate about the safety of one of
> the most heralded interventions in AIDS prevention: use of the drug
> Nevirapine to prevent ... *Science Magazine* Dec 23, 2004

Whistleblower talks of 'poorly conducted' drug study Jan 4, 2005. It involved giving the AIDS drug, Nevirapine to pregnant women to prevent the infection from being transmitted to their babies. *WBOC TV*

Doctors demand immediate access to antiretroviral drugs in Africa

Dr Peter Mugyenyi, director of the Joint Clinical Research Centre in Kampala, Uganda, told the conference, hosted by the centre and convened by the Rockefeller Foundation, that there was "moral outrage" over the continued loss of prime life in Africa when effective drugs existed and were cheap to manufacture. (Annabel Ferriman, *Kampala BMJ 2001;322:1018*, 28 April 2001)

AIDS drugs plan starts in Uganda and Cote d'Ivoire, By Peter Mwaura. *Africa Recovery* Vol 11. Number 3. Page17

BRAZIL'S RIGHT TO SAVE LIVES, New York Times Editorial, June 23, 2005
http://www.nytimes.com/2005/06/23/opinion/23thu3.html

Life: The cost of living, Lifeonline: A multimedia initiative about the effect of globalization.
www.tve.org/lifeonline/index.

ABBOTT LOWERS PRICE OF ANTIRETROVIRAL KALETRA IN BRAZIL; GOVERNMENT DROPS THREAT TO BREAK PATENT, Jul 11, 2005
http://www.kaisernetwork.org/daily_reports/rep_index.

The Global Fund to fight AIDS, tuberculosis and malaria,
www.theglobalfund.org/en/ - 54k - 13 Dec 2006

President's Emergency Plan for AIDS Relief (PEPFAR),
www.avert.org/pepfar.htm

Index